Create A Healthy Heart

I DID IT
WHY DON'T YOU?

by

Narinder K. Saini, MD
Edited by Anne E. Deam

ISBN 0-9654590-0-4

Published by Healthy Heart Publishing
3135 Imperial Blvd.
Springfield, OH 45503

Printed in the United States of America

Designed and produced by
Griffith Publishing Consultants, Caldwell, Idaho

Surya Namaskar illustration by Parakh Saini

*This book is dedicated to my parents,
who believed in me and my mission,
To my dear wife Uma, who supported
me with her endless love,
To my kids—Punam, Monica and
Kavita—who gave me support and
strength.*

**Atherosclerosis
is a disease of choice.
You
can choose
to prevent it.**

Contents

Illustrations and Tables

Foreword

Dr. Saini's work and service has profoundly influenced me and thousands of my patients to lead a healthy and happy lifestyle.

It is always disappointing for an invasive and interventional cardiologist like me to take care of chronic, recurrent and, at times, devastating consequences of coronary artery disease. The enthusiastic and overwhelming support and care in the prevention and regression of coronary artery disease by Dr. Saini result in positive and permanent outcomes for hundreds of patients.

I am also proud of Dr. Saini and his courage to face his own challenge of coronary artery disease, for which he underwent coronary artery bypass surgery, angioplasty and stent placement. When all else failed, he resorted to a prevention and regression program on my advice. He not only follows this program scrupulously but also helps others who are victims of the same problem he has faced. I have read this book, Dr. Saini's first, from beginning to end, and I can say it is a true living story of a warrior of disabling coronary artery disease.

Dr. Saini has become a role model for his patients and colleagues. He is known to be a humanist, a sensitive a caring individual, a physician, a social worker, a good friend, and a person who has touched many people in many ways to improve their lives. His heart and soul are in his book. I hope you will benefit from reading this book as much as I have.

Tajuddin Ahmed, M.D.
Chairman, Section of Cardiology
The Community Hospital of Springfield and Clark County
Associate Clinical Professor of Medicine, Wright State
University School of Medicine

"Out of every Crisis comes the *Chance* to be reborn"—Nena O'Neill

"First I was Dying to Finish High School and Start College,
Then I was Dying to Finish College and Start Working,
Then I was Dying to get Married and have Children,
Then I was Dying for my children to grow old,
Then I was Dying to Retire. . .
. . . And now I am dying and I
Suddenly realized that...*I Forgot to Live*."

Anonymous

Acknowledgments

I want to thank my grandparents, particularly my Nana Jee, who always thought of me being a doctor, because I had a "gentle heart" (his words). I am indebted to my respected father and mother who always believed in me and would always put me at ease when ever I had an unresolved conflict by saying "let the life unfold itself as it is and always trust the Almighty God."

I want to thank my wife, my loving friend who had to go to the kids' recitals and other functions alone when I was too busy doing what I enjoyed most—taking care of patients—the wife who slept on the hospital floor or chair when I was sick in the hospital for six weeks.

I am grateful to my precious kids—Punam, Monica and Kavita (particularly Punam who was not given much attention by me during my residency and who used to be the target of my anger). Without their support and strength I would not have the courage to write this book. I appreciate my dear brothers, Paul, my sisters in law, who were always there for me regardless of anything, and my friends, co-workers and patients in Urbana, Dayton and Springfield, who supported me to write this book to share my experience.

A special word for Liz Mount, a superb dietitian, mother and educator. Without her help I would not have been able to work with my patients to reverse their coronary artery disease. She helped me writing the chapter on healthy eating and collected all the recipes for this book.

As I share with you the concept of creating a healthy heart I am also making a political statement that our medical system is in a total mess. If we, the people, don't take charge of our own health, we are going to be in trouble. As a nation we cannot afford to pay for health care which rewards you only when you are sick. We need to move on from sickness to wellness and fitness. It is better and cheaper this way. I trust that by sharing my experience with you about creating a healthy heart, I can enrich your journey towards total and holistic health.   **Narinder K. Saini**

Introduction

"It is always preferable to have one's face turned towards the Future than towards the Past."

Sri Aurobondo

I wanted to write this book sharing how I suddenly realized that *"I forgot to live"* when I was having serious problems lying in the hospital bed after my angioplasty. I wanted to share what I learned from that experience to let others know how a person is reborn after facing the crisis.

I hope this book will encourage those who are down and depressed after having a serious problem and asking, "Why me?"

I hope this book will encourage them to take their lives in their control and use their power of prevention and prayers to change their lifestyle in the process of creating a healthy heart.

I hope that this book will be read by people who want to learn from the experience of others and take charge of their lives.

I want you, the reader, to understand that your body will forgive the abuses you went through all this time by eating all that grease, by being a couch potato and by stressing your lives to the limit—and will give you a healthy choice to live.

I would like to invite you to read this book as a tool to equip yourself to reverse heart disease or prevent it even if you have not been afflicted. To be technically and anatomically correct, whenever I say "heart disease" I actually mean obstructive CAD (coronary artery disease). CAD means that arteries which supply blood to the heart muscle are plugged up by debris from cholesterol and/or other material. This blocked artery eventually cuts off the blood supply carrying oxygen, an important nutrient for the cells, to that part of the heart muscle. During this process the cells die because the essential nutrient, oxygen, is not supplied, resulting in chest pain and finally heart attack. Remember, whenever I say heart disease I actually mean an obstructive coronary artery disease.

This book is a testament to the connection between mind and body and the power that you have within you to tackle any problems, particularly heart disease. Although the focus is the same for any chronic problem, I would like to share with you my own personal triumph over this deadly disease and similar triumphs of many people who believed in me and in themselves.

The following scene is very common on such popular TV series as "E.R," "Chicago Hope" and others:

"Everybody clear!" screams a doctor or a nurse. Defibrillator paddles are placed on the chest of a patient who has had a cardiac arrest (which means that the heart has stopped pumping). One of two things will happen to the patient: a normal heart rhythm will be restored, or the patient will die. After the TV shoot, the actor or actress who has suffered a "cardiac arrest" gets up and goes on to other things.

In real life, however, all too often the patient dies. That's exactly what almost happened to me in early 1991 when I was going through the procedure of angioplasty to open up one of my obstructed coronary arteries. Because my rhythm disturbance was not that life threatening, I was lucky enough to survive and write about my experience to **create a healthy heart** for myself. I offer a challenge: **If I did it, why don't you?**

Things in my life have never come easily, and I am not professing that it will be easy for you, either. But if you can trust yourself and listen to "the little you" inside known as our conscience, the part of you that tells you that nobody else, only you can take care of yourself, you can **create a healthy heart** for yourself.

We as physicians now know and accept that we can do only so much; ultimately you are the one who is respon-sible for your own health. If we all do our share of creating a **Healthy Heart,** then and then only can we tackle this monstrous problem of our nation known as the HEALTH CARE CRISIS.

You know and I know that health care in the USA is so costly that one can no longer afford to get sick. Although we are the richest nation in the world, the cost of the health care is almost bankrupting our nation. We are spending too much money for at least one disease which is preventable. Fifty percent of premature death is preventable, twenty percent is the result of genetic factors, and twenty percent is due to environmental factors and the remaining ten percent comes from other factors.

Heart disease ranks first in deaths in the United States. But does it have to? Do people have to die from heart disease? Do people have to fall prey to heart disease in the first place? If your parents or grandparents had heart disease, are you doomed to have it, too? Is a genetic factor alone enough to include your name in the obituary column? The answer to all of the above questions is: *maybe not.*

As a physician, I was used to dealing with other people's illnesses, including heart disease. I had seen the ravages of heart disease in others. Was I prepared for heart disease to impact my own life? And at age 42? Absolutely not. I was shocked when I was diagnosed as having heart disease. I had no family history of heart disease or other contributing factors such as high blood pressure, smoking or a high cholesterol level.

Did I learn anything from this experience? Plenty. I learned that a low-fat diet, exercise, stress management and proper medications can prevent or reverse the course of heart disease. By sharing this information, can I help others prevent heart disease or reverse the coronary artery disease that has already occurred? **I believe so.**

What I want to share with you is not a doctor-to-patient lecture. I want to share with you what I have learned as a patient who almost died from heart disease. What I have learned is even more amazing than the fact that I survived when so many people have died. What I have learned is **how to *prevent* heart disease** or, as in my case and others, **how to *reverse* the coronary artery disease** that already has begun. I want to share the missing link that I and the medical community were really not aware of until the late 80s and early 90s.

From my studies, personal experience, my patients, and discussions with other experts, I have learned that a healthy heart, either through prevention or reversal of coronary artery disease, rests upon what I term the **three pillars of life: stress management, exercise,** and **diet.** Through ongoing studies with patients in a cardiac prevention and rehabilitation program, I have found that proper exercise, diet, and stress management not only can drastically reduce a person's risk of heart disease, but also reverse the progress of coronary artery disease.

In this book I will explain to you the importance of stress management, exercise, and diet and how to take control of them in your life. I also will discuss other important issues relating to your heart. I will tell you what you need to do to keep your heart healthy, or to reverse the coronary artery disease that may already have begun. As a result of my personal experience with heart disease, I can share with you first hand how stress management, exercise and diet can prevent and reverse coronary artery disease and how these measures prevent the need for surgery and other invasive procedures. I speak first as a former patient and then as a physician—a patient who has been able to make these changes, and a doctor who knows you can, too.

In order to have a healthy heart, you must follow the guidelines for stress management, aerobic exercise, and a low fat diet. I always tell my patients that I am not here to prolong their lives, but to help them live healthier, improve their quality of life and prepare for more enjoyable lives without the suffering that so often accompanies the end of life. In reality, it is the quality of life which is important and not the longevity.

For patients diagnosed with an obstructive coronary artery disease the normal run-of-the-mill medical wisdom is to send the patient either for an open heart surgery or to an expert cardiologist who could open up the artery by angioplasty. This procedure of angioplasty is done by newer techniques now using drillers, stretchers, scrapers, lasers and stents. But let me share with you a third **not commonly prescribed** mode of treatment which is known as "Reversal of Coronary Artery Disease by Life Style Changes." I am by no means suggesting that if you are having an emergency or life threatening heart disease you should opt for this mode of treatment. In an emergency, you need emergency procedures. This mode of treatment is for those people only who are ready to commit themselves to lifelong positive changes toward a more healthy and accepting lifestyle. These lifestyle changes can be incorporated before or after a heart attack, bypass surgery or angioplasty.

Not in competition with Western medicine, I am suggesting complementing it with alternative medicine, in combination with heart-healthy lifestyle changes. As you will see, heart disease is a disease of lifestyle. If one's lifestyle is successfully changed, the ravages of heart disease, for the most part, can be dramatically altered or prevented before they have occurred.

Let me make it clear that Western medicine has made wonderful progress. The advances in the last century are unparalleled. We can do so much with the diseases of our body that was never dreamed of. All the progress made in treating infectious diseases and the surgical marvel of doing bypass, transplants and the astronomical diagnostic jumps we have been able to make can only be humbly respected. But in that progress, where the emphasis and concentration was placed on the body and the body only, we lost millennia of valuable research done by our ancestors on the power of mind in preventing or curing diseases. We concentrated so much on the body that we lost the connection between mind and body. The time has come to join the mind and the body again. I have found this to be true in my research. In the chapters that follow I will discuss the mind and body connection as it was so nicely presented by pioneer of mind body connection, Deepak Chopra M.D, as well as the necessary lifestyle changes that need to be made and other topics relevant to a healthy heart.

To give you a complete understanding of the personal discoveries that I have made, I will begin my story when I first became aware of heart disease in my life. I am convinced that stress played a major role in that and I will relate to you how stress, lack of exercise, and a poor diet resulted in my own heart disease. I will share with you how heart disease awakened me and challenged me to take control of my life, to make wise decisions and permanent changes, and to set new goals that led me to a healthier lifestyle. Finally, because I have been able to change, you will learn that you, too, can make these changes to have a healthy heart.

I will never forget the time a female patient told me about the pain associated with childbirth as being the worst pain a woman could ever have. I remarked that I knew it was very painful. She smiled and replied, "How would you know? You have never been through that experience." And she was right. The pain of childbirth is one pain that I will never know. However, I know the pain of heart disease; I experienced it firsthand and saw its effects on my family and friends. On the subject of heart disease, I can speak with authority. It is the authority born of experience.

Today we are dealing with many diseases of choice, not of chance. Half of our diseases are preventable. I know some CEOs who make and manage million-dollar deals and are good at making their financial portfolios and those of others prosper but are very poor in managing their own health portfolio. We all need to make a sound financial and health portfolio, and you are better off if you become manager of your own health. Your good health is too precious to be entrusted to the doctors only.

However, before I begin my personal story, let me explain to you what coronary artery disease is, and what we know about it.

1

What Is Coronary Artery Disease?

"The story's about you."—Horace (65-8 BC)

WORDS WE USE IN MEDICINE TO REFER TO THE heart generally come from the Greek words "myo" for muscle and "kardio" for heart. The heart is a muscle that pumps five or more quarts of blood throughout the circulatory system in the lapse of a minute. It pumps about two thousand gallons of blood every day.

The heart itself is really two muscles or two pumps, each consisting of two chambers. When these muscles contract or squeeze together, blood flows from the upper chamber, or atrium, to the lower chamber, or ventricle. The chambers are connected by a series of valves. The blood enters the right atrium through the superior vena cava, from the upper part of the body, the inferior vena cava, from the lower part of the body, and from the coronary sinus which drains blood from the heart muscle. The blood then flows from the right atrium through the tricuspid valve into the right ventricle and is ejected by rhythmic, synchronous contractions of the heart muscle, through the pulmonary valve into the pulmonary artery to the lungs where carbon dioxide is removed.

Oxygen-enriched blood returns from the lungs via pulmonary veins. It passes from the left atrium through the mitral valve into the left ventricle and then exits through the aortic valve into the aorta to be circulated to the body's organs and extremities. The right and left sides of the heart contract and relax simultaneously. The heart rate varies, depending on the body's level of exertion.

The right and left coronary arteries originate from the aorta, the largest blood vessel in the body, and branch off to supply blood to all areas of the heart: external and internal surfaces and cardiac tissue. Coronary artery disease (CAD) is characterized by narrowing or obstruction in the interior walls of the coronary arteries, and one or more of the arteries may eventually become completely blocked.

This narrowing or obstruction interferes with, restricts, or if the artery is completely blocked, prohibits blood flow to the heart muscle; therefore, when the heart does not receive an adequate supply of blood and oxygen to nourish itself, cardiac problems occur. As a result of the insufficient blood supply, certain diseases may develop such as angina pectoris, a constricting pain in the chest; congestive heart failure, the heart's inability to pump an adequate blood and oxygen supply resulting in a surplus of fluid around the heart and other organs which creates other complications; or abnormal heart rhythms which can lead to sudden cardiac death.

Coronary artery disease results from atherosclerosis, a type of arteriosclerosis, or hardening of the arteries. Hardening of the coronary arteries primarily occurs in the arteries on the heart's surface. Atherosclerosis develops slowly from childhood and progresses throughout life. Symptoms of the disease generally appear in middle age or later in life when the heart's blood supply is not adequate to meet its needs.

Degenerative changes, or changes marked by deterioration, occur within the walls of the artery. Plaque, a hard sticky substance, develops within and beneath the blood vessel's inner layer. This lipid or fatty debris is comprised mainly of cholesterol derived from low density lipoproteins (LDL, bad cholesterol) as well as triglycerides and phospholipids.

These lipid or fatty deposits, or atheromas, as they are called, are found near areas of turbulent blood flow where the artery's diameter decreases and arteries fork into branches. As the blood flow increases in blood vessels with a decreased diameter, the resulting elevated pressure inside the artery enhances the formation of plaque.

Coronary arteries are particularly vulnerable to atherosclerosis or hardening as a result of a decrease in the heart's oxygen supply due to a lack of supplementary or secondary blood supply. Atherosclerosis impedes the blood flow because of plaque buildup in the arteries, blood clots which form around plaque, hemorrhages or bleeding in damaged walls of blood vessels, and hardened arteries which do not dilate properly.

Many different theories try to explain why plaque forms in the first place. All the theories relating to plaque suggest that the lining of the artery undergoes change and that LDL cholesterol infiltrates the lining of the blood vessel. In the final stage, plaque hardens and sometimes breaks loose resulting in a blood clot.

The inner lining of the artery is actually as smooth as glass and permits two thousand gallons of blood to pass through each day. The blood carries oxygen in the red blood cells to the three trillion cells in the body. The inside lining of the artery is covered by HDL (good) cholesterol. This cholesterol acts like a lubricant so that the blood can pass through the artery without any delay. If for some reason the inner side of the artery is not as smooth or because of toxic stress or toxic chemicals, there is injury to the inside of the artery. Platelets, also called the cement of the body, will deposit at the site of the injury. This mechanism is similar to what happens when you have an external cut or injury to the skin where the blood clots, forming an irregular surface. The same sequence of events happening inside the arterial wall will allow cholesterol and other material to deposit, slowly forming and obstructing the artery. The theory is not so simple as it sounds, and the injury goes through multiple biochemical changes to form an atheroma.

Since a person can have coronary atherosclerosis or hardening of the arteries for years without any outward sign, understanding the risk factors is essential. One *major* risk factor in conjunction with one or more *contributing* risk factors places a person at a high risk of developing coronary artery disease.

Contributing risk factors

Heredity

A family history of coronary artery disease increases the risk of developing coronary artery disease.

Gender

More men than women develop coronary artery disease. Men develop it at an earlier age. However, after menopause, women become as likely as men to develop coronary artery disease.

Race

Black women of all ages and black men under 45 have an increased incidence of hypertension (high blood pressure), which increases the risk for coronary artery disease.

Age

The death rate from coronary artery disease increases with age.

These contributing factors cannot be changed. However, other major risk factors are controllable:

Major risk factors

High blood pressure

Hypertension or high blood pressure leads to atherosclerosis or hardening of the arteries. The higher the pressure, the greater the chance of developing coronary artery disease. However, even a moderate pressure increase can lead to coronary artery disease if a person has other risk factors.

Hypertension frequently affects people who are middle aged and elderly, blacks, those who have a heavy alcohol intake, and women who use oral contraceptives. Diabetics and those who suffer from gout may also be hypertensive.

Although the relationship is not completely understood, some studies suggest that elevated blood pressure damages the lining of blood vessels.

Smoking

A person who smokes a pack of cigarettes daily is more than twice as likely to develop coronary artery disease than a nonsmoker. A person who smokes two packs a day is four times as likely to develop it. However, people who successfully quit smoking eventually return to the same risk level as the nonsmoker.

Smoking has a detrimental effect on blood vessels because inhaled nicotine constricts them. Nicotine also promotes blood clots because it neutralizes the body's anticoagulant, or anti-clot forming compound, heparin. Smoking stimulates the collection of platelets and releases chemicals that cause blood vessels to spasm. Smoking increases catecholamine levels which speed the heart rate, elevate blood pressure, and irritate the lining of blood vessels.

In addition, smoking promotes abnormal heart rhythms and decreases lung capacity. It also reduces the body's level of Vitamin C which helps to metabolize cholesterol.

Elevated blood cholesterol

Cholesterol itself is not bad. The body produces cholesterol, which is used in hormone regulation and other bodily processes. However, the risk of coronary artery disease increases when blood cholesterol levels exceed 200 mg/dl. Too much cholesterol, particularly the LDL cholesterol component, can damage the arteries, leading to accelerated atherosclerosis. A high cholesterol level in conjunction with high blood pressure worsens the effect on blood vessels.

Cholesterol travels in lipoprotein complexes in the bloodstream. Many factors determine the rate at which cholesterol leaves the interior walls of blood vessels. They are diet, genetic factors, the ratio of HDL (good cholesterol) to total cholesterol, and blood vessel pressure. Until the age of women's menopause, more men than women have abnormally high cholesterol levels.

Diabetes

Male diabetics are twice as likely to develop coronary artery disease than non-diabetics, and women with diabetes are three times as likely to develop it. Many diabetics have decreased HDL levels, increased platelet adhesions, and other blood clotting abnormalities. A high level of glucose may cause sugar to deposit on the arterial walls.

Elevated triglycerides

The risk of coronary artery disease doubles when serum triglycerides exceed 200 mg/dl. Triglycerides may pick up extra amounts of Apoliprotein E and bind with LDL (bad cholesterol) receptors which enter the walls of arteries and lead to cholesterol deposits. A high trigliceride level is a known risk factor for women.

Obesity

High blood pressure and a high level of total cholesterol in an obese person increase the risk for CAD. When an obese person with high blood pressure and high cholesterol levels loses weight, both blood pressure and LDL cholesterol levels decrease. Adults who are obese have a greater chance of developing diabetes, which also increases the risk for coronary artery disease.

Lack of exercise

Inactivity increases the level of LDL (bad cholesterol). Atherosclerosis progresses more rapidly in inactive people. Regular exercise increases HDL cholesterol levels, lowers resting heart rate, lowers LDL cholesterol and improves oxygenation of the heart. Aerobic exercise improves oxygen extraction from the blood while minimally elevating diastolic pressure (pressure of the resting heart). Anaerobic exercise dramatically increases blood pressure, which may lead to angina and abnormal heart rhythms. See Chapter 9 for more on exercise and healthy hearts.

Stress

Stress increases levels of circulating catecholamines which increase blood pressure and the consumption of oxygen by the heart. Stress can lead to overeating, fatigue, lack of exercise, and abnormal heart rhythms. A Type A personality has twice the normal risk of coronary artery disease in both youth and middle age. The Type A personality exhibits a chronic overreaction to stress, excessive aggressiveness, greater competitiveness, and hostility.

Do you know that women who talk on the phone more than five times a day live longer compare with females calling less than two times a day? It is also scientifically recognized now that there is healing power of prayer.

Coronary artery disease is the result of a combination of controllable and uncontrollable factors. However, coronary artery disease can be prevented before it has begun. It can also be reversed, and its progression can be stopped.

Out of seven major modifiable risk factors, four of them depend on the patient's lifestyle:

Stress
Smoking
Obesity
Lack of exercise

The other three are *influenced* by lifestyle:

Hypertension

Abnormal lipids

Diabetes

In the next chapter, I will share with what I learned from my own experience with heart disease and explain why, in reality, heart disease does not have to be the Number One cause of death in the United States.

2

Stressed Into Heart Disease

"It is bad to have an empty purse, but an empty heart is a whole lot worse."—Nixon Waterman

WHAT IS STRESS, ANYWAY? DOESN'T EVERYONE have stress in daily life? Stress has been a buzzword for several decades. It is today nearly impossible to pick up a magazine, newspaper, or book on health without seeing the word "stress." In the early 1980s, stress was linked to burnout on the job. Stress and job were inextricably bound together.

In the 1990s, stress and health have come to the forefront. Not only do we know that stress is physically as well as psychologically harmful, we have also learned that stress alone or when combined with other risk factors can be fatal. However, it is not *stress* itself which is a killer; it is the manner in which a person *handles* stress that has become a key to unraveling the mystery behind heart disease.

As a physician I became acutely aware of feeling stressed in my practice around 1987. By 1989, I had become disenchanted with the medical profession. No longer was I the sole judge of a patient's condition or treatment. The art of practicing medicine was taken over by a person sitting at a computer, making critical decisions on the telephone miles away to allow or refuse treatment for patients. Physician-oriented medicine had become "remote control medicine."

The healing process, involving touching and sharing, was replaced by HMOs, whose sole purpose is to make money, and others whose interests were focused on saving dollars. They were making decisions that only the attending physician should have been making. I am not saying that physicians were not responsible, in part, for the demise in the way medicine was formerly practiced; however, I was not trained to practice medicine the "new" way, and I found it very frustrating to have lost control of patient care.

In my practice I realized that I was spending less time with my patients and more time with paperwork. Instead of encouraging my patients to come with written questions and spending ample time with them as had been my custom, I was hurrying patients through their appointments as a result of calls from insurance companies nurses and company physicians who review procedures for insurance companies. The appointment time my patients were paying for were partially consumed by the administrative duties I was being forced to perform for the insurance companies. As a result, I became distressed and depressed over changes in the practice of medicine and my inability to control those outside factors. I would go home depressed knowing that I had hurried some of my patients and possibly did not answer all of their questions. Almost every evening I would tell my wife that I was no longer enjoying my medical practice and that the guilt of not giving my one hundred percent to my patients was bothering me.

Although none of my patients had ever complained to me about the decreasing amount of time that I spent with them, I knew that the quality of patient care was not the same as I was used to providing them two or three years previously.

My inability to care for patients the way that I knew I should made me feel **guilty**. Sometimes I would sleep poorly because of the guilt and sometimes the following morning I would call some of the previous day's patients to see if I had answered their questions.

In addition, a hectic schedule at the hospital where I was chief of medical staff began to take its toll. My office staff and family members who were my best friends told me to slow down as they saw how distressed I was. To compensate for my lack of time, the staff spent more time with my patients to answer their questions and tried to be a good buffer for me.

Medicine had become stressful rather than pleasurable as it once had been. Retrospectively I think that my main problem was that I did not know how to handle stress. Money had never been a driving force for me. I used to say that if I worked hard, my patients would pay me; if I did not work hard, they would not pay me. I appreciated the fact that they always thought that I deserved to be paid.

In December 1989, a friend from India who came to visit me was shocked to see that I had gained about twenty pounds. He brought to my attention the problems that I had neglected regarding my own health. Trying to take care of my patients and adapt to a changing medical profession, I had failed to take care of myself.

My friend's look of surprise at my weight gain focused my attention on what I had not been doing in my personal life. I was not eating right and I was not exercising. It seemed as though I did not have enough time to eat right because I was always rushing around. I acted as if nothing harmful could ever happen to me.

My friend encouraged me to start exercising; when he left town, I decided to begin exercising regularly. I played racquetball a few times and realized how out of shape I had become. After a couple minutes of play, I found my heart had raced from 90 to 150 beats per minute, and I was short of breath.

I followed the advice I had given to hundreds of my patients over the age of forty: to have a cardiovascular stress test before beginning any intensive exercise program. During the stress test, a patient is hooked up to an electrocardiogram (EKG) monitor while walking on a treadmill. The patient is stressed physically on the treadmill to reach a prescribed target heart rate which is different for different age groups. A physician is present to note any abnormal changes in the EKG and any abnormal blood pressure response as the speed and angle of elevation of the treadmill are increased. My stress test showed some questionable changes in the EKG which were considered abnormal in comparison with my previous EKGs, and I was told to repeat the test in six months.

After thinking about what I would have recommended to my patients, I opted to have further testing without delay. I decided to have a stress thallium, which is more extensive than a stress test. In a stress thallium test, the patient walks on a treadmill to elevate the heart rate as you would normally do in the simple stress test, but once the heart rate has been elevated to the prescribed level, an injection of thallium, a radioactive tracer used in scintillation or fluorescent scanning, is injected into the patient's vein. The patient continues walking on the treadmill for at least another minute after the injection. Then, the patient's heart is scanned by a machine similar to an X-ray machine, and the blood flow through the coronary arteries is filmed for later study by a specialist. About two to three hours later, the patient returns for further scanning which monitors blood flow through the coronary arteries while the heart is at rest.

My stress thallium results, like those of the stress test, indicated questionable changes or differences from those obtained on a prior EKG. With no family history of heart disease and no visible risk factors, I was told that I could repeat the test in six months.

At that time, a good friend and cardiologist, Dr. Tajuddin Ahmed, advised me to have a spectrum thallium stress test done. This test was capable of producing more detailed images than those provided by other gamma cameras. It increased the diagnostic accuracy from 80 to 90 percent. My Spectrum Thallium results showed some obstructed arteries. Dr. Ahmed and I agreed that I should undergo a cardiac catheterization to make sure that we were not overlooking a serious problem. The cardiac catheterization was scheduled for a Friday in an out-of-town hospital, and I had every intention of returning to work the following Monday.

Early the next morning, my wife, my brother, and I, who had not eaten breakfast, went to the hospital. We sat in the waiting room until I was called to the patient registration area to give them the needed insurance information. Knowing that I was a physician, the person to whom I gave my insurance card, a woman in her forties, asked me how to lose weight. She was overweight and had difficulty breathing. I told her to exercise and to eat the right kind of food. I informed her that I was in the hospital to have a cardiac procedure because I had failed to do those two things: eat right and exercise. She replied that she had difficulty exercising and eating right because she loved to eat and hated to exercise. I did not respond, but I thought to myself, "That is what we all say." Isn't that the truth?

If I could prescribe exercise in a capsule I could become an instant millionaire. (I am working on it.)

After finishing the registration procedure, I was admitted to the hospital. In preparation for the cardiac catheterization, a nurse started an intravenous (IV) line to give me fluids and medications, and then I was taken to the cardiac catheter lab. About fifteen minutes later, the doctor arrived and started the procedure on time. The doctor inserted the catheter into my groin and instructed the x-ray technician to be ready to start taking pictures of the arteries when he injected the dye.

As I watched the procedure on a monitor, I saw an obstruction in the first artery the physician injected. The second and third arteries were also obstructed. No one in the lab said a word. I broke the silence "I think that I need to have bypass surgery," I said. The cardiologist who had been quiet till now told me that there was a problem that needed to be remedied. With my permission, he called a good friend of mine who is a cardiothoracic surgeon to come to evaluate the problem. Immediately he came to see me and concurred with our decision. It was decided that I should have emergency bypass surgery without delay, not even a trip home.

As the result of all this unexpected commotion, I began to have some chest pain, which was treated promptly by those wonderful nurses with the prescribed medications. In the meantime the surgeon and cardiologist went out and talked with my wife about my need for bypass surgery. You can imagine how upset she was because till now I was telling her that everything was going to be fine.

It was a shock to all of us—my wife, my brother, and my whole family—but there was no other alternative at that time because during those days the only way we knew how to treat this type of heart disease was either by surgery or by balloon angioplasty. Once the decision was made to have bypass surgery, I called my office staff to inform them of the problem. We worked out a sensible solution of how to provide care to my patients for the next couple of weeks. To this day I am thankful to them for the job well done.

The next step was to obtain coverage of my practice while I was in the hospital. With the help of my office staff, we were able to enlist three physicians to cover for me. Because I was chief of medical staff, I asked the administrator of the hospital to arrange for coverage of those duties as well.

The following day, with lots of emotional support from my family that included my wife and my brothers, staff and friends, I had my bypass surgery. I felt lucky because I had attacked the disease before it had attacked me.

After surgery, I remembered waking up and seeing tubes all over me; I was unable to speak because of a tube in my mouth. I was able to communicate with my wife through sign language although I was not very good at it. The first thing that I told her was that I was thankful to the Good Lord to be alive and to have made it through surgery.

My wife, who was and still is a great support and comfort to me, was able to take me home on the fifth day. In

1989, being able to go home on the fifth day was excellent. In 1996, going home on the fourth or fifth day is standard protocol. Before leaving the hospital, I was told to exercise, eat right, and take care of myself, a 30-second prescription which takes me about an hour or so to prescribe now.

Before going home I was told by the floor nurses that two of my patients had been admitted on the same floor of the hospital to have bypass surgery that week. As a newly discharged patient, I decided to make rounds to see those two patients and encourage them personally and answer any questions they had. When you are going through a major surgery like this, a little encouragement from a patient who already has gone through this can really help you. I just wanted to tell them that there is nothing to it. They were surprised and of course happy to see me. One of the patients, who was reluctant to have bypass surgery, was relieved when he saw me. Although he was the president of a bank, he had a difficult time coming to terms with the idea of bypass surgery. My visit with him made him very happy and later on he had a very successful and uneventful surgery. At the end of my rounds, I walked to the intensive care unit and thanked the staff for their help and excellent work.

Within two weeks, I was working at the office part-time; within four weeks, I was working full-time. I felt a strong sense of commitment to my patients, some of whom were older and did not want to go to see any other doctor. I started to enjoy my practice again, but soon the stress returned. I found myself fighting with insurance companies over procedures and admissions of my patients in the hospital for proper observation and treatment, rushing through my schedule, and slowly getting into the same stressful situations again.

Six months after surgery, I was doing fine and was very active in my practice again. One fine morning I was informed that a young patient of mine had gone to the emergency room with chest pain, but his insurance company plan would not let him be admitted because he did not have any acute changes in his EKG. That means that the EKG (which is tracing of electrical impulses recorded from the heart on the paper) was not showing an impending or recent heart attack and the blood work, etc. was OK. Although his tests were normal, after seeing him in the emergency room myself and knowing about his very strong family history of premature heart disease, I called the insurance company, asking them to grant me permission to admit and observe him.

The insurance company refused to give me permission to admit him to the hospital because he did not meet the company's criteria for admission. The hospital was kind enough to agree with me not to charge the patient for the stay, and I told the insurance company that I was not going to charge them either for this admission. In spite of this I was not able to convince them to let me observe the patient in the hospital and had to let him go against medical advice.

I wasted half a day of my time on the phone being put on hold even before I could explain to the operator why I was calling. I kept thinking about my patients, who had been waiting for an hour. I knew that when I went back I was going to have to rush through my schedule. That guilt and stress were enough to raise my heart rate and blood pressure; I remember I was ready to throw in the towel. But worrying about my wonderful patients kept me going. Money was never an attraction for me but their smiling faces, loves and hugs would make me forget all my anger and frustrations.

Later that night, the patient returned to the hospital with a massive heart attack. He survived, but I wondered if I could have changed the course of events had he been permitted to stay in the hospital earlier in the day. I started wondering how many people this method of practicing medicine by remote control, would admit to hospitals when it was too late. The writing was on the wall. It seemed the only way medicine would be practiced any more. I said to myself, "if you cannot fit into this new wave of *for profit health care system* then you'd better get out."

Stressed and upset, I began to wonder if I wanted to practice medicine in this manner. I had had enough; this incident was enough to make me cry. I was trained like so many other physicians to be an honest and caring person whose whole responsibility was to care for and provide patients with the medical wisdom to relieve them from the misery of disease. My sacred oath expected me to do that, but more and more I was feeling a misfit in this new wave of healthcare. I am not in any way defending a few of my greedy colleagues. There are always a black sheep in any profession, but most are caring individuals.

I had the responsibility for twenty-five hundred patients, two thousand of whom were older patients on Medicare. I say "responsibility" because when patients choose a doctor they are basically asking you to help them deal with the diseases they may have. It then becomes my responsibility to provide them with the art of medicine I was trained for. I found myself in the same precarious position—not enough time for my patients, and the situation was getting worse. I had not been able to accept any new patients for four to five years.

One day at home, while having a conversation about a personal matter, I became upset and started having chest pain. I went to the hospital for an EKG, which, much to my surprise, showed some changes. Another cardiac catheterization revealed that all except one of my bypass grafts were blocked, all within a year of bypass surgery. Depressed and upset, I wondered, "Why me? Where did I go wrong?" It appeared that I would have to have bypass surgery again, but we decided to try angioplasty first on the original arteries where the blockage was at the same location as before.

My good friend and cardiologist recommended that I go to Emory Hospital in Atlanta. This hospital performed the first angioplasty in the USA by a pioneer cardiologist Dr. Grundig, a procedure in which an inflated balloon at the end of a catheter pushes built-up plaque against the walls of the artery, compressing the plaque and opening the closure of the artery, allowing the blood to flow freely through the artery.

The morning before I left home for Atlanta, I celebrated my birthday with my family and friends. All my friends came to celebrate with me and to wish me good luck. After the party, my wife and my brother went with me to Atlanta for moral support.

The procedure began on time. The physician asked me if I wanted to watch the angioplasty on a screen that was in the room. I saw the first artery being slowly ballooned out as the balloon was inflated; this part of the procedure took only five minutes. The artery was almost one hundred percent open. However, problems developed getting the catheter into the second artery. When the catheter was in place and the balloon inflated, the artery tore under the pressure of forcing it open. After unsuccessfully trying to repair the artery, the doctor inserted a stent, which is like a coil, to keep the artery open. After six hours on the table, I was sent to the intensive care unit.

Following the angioplasty, I was instructed to lie flat in bed to prevent any movement which would trigger bleeding. I was given blood thinner and, after twenty-four hours, I was moved to another room. The second day I experienced some chest pain that subsided a while later. I had the feeling that something had gone wrong, but the EKG was normal. After the third or fourth day, I noticed blood in my urine. The doctor assured me that sometimes blood can appear in urine because of the blood thinner I was getting and told me not to worry. On the seventh or eighth day, I was more stable but still had some blood in my urine. I was released from the hospital and flew home with my family. All this time I was in the hospital, my wife slept on the floor and on a couch in my room, and for a few days, my brother slept in a nearby hotel room.

I can't forget the misery I put them through. For the last twenty years of my practice I have noticed that if the male spouse is sick, the wife will be there for him all the time, but unfortunately, the reverse is not true. Even now in our cardiac rehabilitation support group the observation is the same. Lately I have noticed that young working female spouses are not as supportive as their older counterparts are. I am not saying this is right or wrong, but I do know that patients who have unconditional support from their spouses and other family members heal better and faster.

I flew home the same day I was discharged. The flight was uneventful except it felt odd sitting and being pushed in a wheelchair by my beautiful wife (male ego, I guess) at the airport. Jenny, my office nurse, brought us home from the airport and I had nice quiet dinner with my family. You can imagine how happy I was in my own castle eating home cooked food and not that nasty hospital food. About 9 o'clock that evening I began to have terrible stomach cramps and vomiting. Not sure what had happened, I was worried that I was having a heart attack. I told my wife that I needed to go to the hospital. A physician friend who came to see me agreed and accompanied me to the hospital in the ambulance.

In the emergency room after ruling out an impending heart attack, doctors shifted the focus to finding other causes of the pain including appendicitis and kidney stones. An x-ray of the kidney revealed a blockage in one of the ureters, the tube that carries urine from the kidney to the bladder. The ureter was blocked by a blood clot, probably caused by an extended period of sitting during the flight home. I was in a great pain. That same night I was admitted to the intensive care unit for observation. The following morning I was pale and anemic. Later on we found out that I had lost three to four pints of blood and was anemic because of the sudden blood loss around the kidney.

After several blood transfusions, I was transferred to the Ohio State University Hospital where initially surgery was planned to unblock the ureter by removing the blood clot. As I had bled into the back of the kidney and was still recovering from angioplasty, the physician opted not to perform the surgery. He hoped that the clot would dissolve itself because the kidney releases an enzyme, urokinase, which acts like a clot buster. I was given morphine injections to help alleviate the pain. As usual I gathered quite a few stories to share with others about the follies in the hospital and about the hospital food, which I can still smell. I may need to write a whole book on this topic!

After a few days, one morning I noticed a change in the color of my urine. My prayers had been answered. The clot was dissolving. The process of healing occurred slowly as the clot dissolved naturally. Finally I began to feel better.

After two weeks more recuperating and a total of six weeks in hospitals, I realized my outlook toward life had changed completely.

One day while sitting in the hospital waiting room, I felt alone, very depressed, and wondered, "Why me, God?" A young girl came and sat down next to me. She looked at me and said, "You are very sad."

I told her that I had been in hospitals for the last six weeks and that I was tired of being sick. At first she smiled; then she started laughing. She had a wonderful smile. Her charming little smile forced me to listen to her. She started explaining to me that she also had been sick and had been battling leukemia for five years. Often she had to go to the hospital for chemotherapy. She stated that during her last stay in the hospital the doctors thought she would die. She had proved them to be wrong and made it because she trusted in the good Lord and had a positive attitude.

She once heard in her church that if you are positive and happy you can kill those bad and ugly cancer cells and that is how she has been fighting this deadly disease by her positive attitude. As we kept on discussing our diseases, she made humorous comments about the nurses. I was struck by her innocence. She asked me to play tic-tac-toe with her, and I played for about an hour until my wife came with some food for me.

The little girl encouraged me to have a positive attitude, keep smiling, and trust that God would take care of me. She told me that if I was sad, I would make others sad, too. She shared with me her secret of success: keep good thoughts, keep smiling, be happy, **be positive** and trust God to know what is best.

Sometimes in your life you meet people who cross your path and make an everlasting impact on your faith in humanity. This girl was a great inspiration for me and made profound changes in my life. She gave me courage to fight when I was depressed and was trying to find the meaning of life. I kept in touch with the little girl until she died a couple of years later, peacefully and on her terms. She will always have a special place in my heart.

3

Awakened to change

"Out of every crisis comes the chance to be reborn."—Nena O'Neill

"BE POSITIVE." THESE ARE TWO LITTLE WORDS but so powerful. When I became aware of the power of faith and trust in the healing process I felt as if someone had given me a new meaning of life. I thought about how the clot in my kidney had dissolved without medicine or surgical intervention.

Being in bed in the hospital and trying to find peace and a reasonable explanation of "why me?" I read quite a few books on different subjects. One book that really hit home was a simple but controversial book written by Dr. Dean Ornish in 1989. He wrote about reversing heart disease with lifestyle changes. I became engrossed in the book. I realized that this is what I needed to do to help myself. This book changed my perception about how I and my colleagues were dealing with the heart disease. In addition, I discovered what I wanted to do with the rest of my life.

You could say that this was a matter of coincidence that I read the book and met the inspiring little girl almost at the same time, but I think that there was a divine intervention that led me to follow a new path of healing. When I returned home from the hospital, I sat down with my family and discussed my new mission.

I decided to do some research on mind and body healing to see if I could help myself and others from this deadly heart disease, and to discover if I could duplicate what was done by pioneer researchers such as Dean Ornish. I wrote letters to my patients about my intention to leave my practice because I was determined not to go through the second open heart surgery as I was recommended to do. I felt that the metaphor for doing the surgery without taking care of the basic problem was just like mopping up the floor without closing a running faucet. For me the running faucet included ignoring stress, eating fatty food, smoking and not exercising regularly. I wanted to prove to myself that I could reverse my obstructive artery disease before I could help somebody else to do so. That meant that I had to quit practicing medicine and begin to practice the regimen outlined for the medical community and the general public by Dean Ornish, and that is exactly what I chose to do.

I knew that practicing remote-controlled medicine was not for me any more, and I wanted to seek alternative ways of helping others and myself to live better. With the approval of my family members, who were unconditionally ready to support me in my mission, I sent out about three thousand letters to my patients explaining to them my intention and reason for stopping my active medical practice and asking for their support, strength and prayers for this new mission. My patients were supportive of my plans and were actually happy for me. I don't think I could have done this without their blessings. I had such a heartening response from them that I told my wife, Uma, a couple of times, "Even if I die today I don't care." When you die you don't take any money and or any materialistic objects with you. The only things that matter are the love, affection and memories which money cannot buy. I am so lucky to be blessed with all of these from such great friends and patients.

With the vision of Dr. Dean Ornish and thanks to the support and faith of the Community Hospital, Springfield, Ohio, and my good friend, Dr. Tajuddin Ahmed, I started a new program at the Coronary Prevention and Rehabilitation Center in Springfield, Ohio, in 1991.

I was convinced that cholesterol was not the whole story; on the contrary, I felt that heart disease is like a mosaic. There are maybe two hundred different risk factors for heart disease. Some of which—such as three Gs: genes, geriatrics and gender—we cannot change. However, we can change other factors such as diet, exercise and managing stress by lifestyle changes.

I wanted to establish a program for patients who had had bypass surgery, heart attacks, angioplasty and for others who wanted to prevent or reverse heart disease. I wanted to give them an alternative which I was not offered and which is still not readily offered. If there is one positive thing I could say about HMOs it is that they are bringing the awareness of prevention in medical practice. Since 1991, I have been involved in the care of more then three thousand patients who had heart disease. In the program we have been able to make healthy changes in their lives. Even if I cannot change every person, each person who does change can influence another person to change. And so the process for change begins and spreads. Perhaps, on a one-to-one basis, we can begin to solve the problem of heart disease in the United States.

We all know that it is very costly to get sick; we cannot afford to get sick. As a nation, we cannot afford to pay the price of treating a disease when prevention is an easier, safer, and a more cost efficient solution.

With the help of a dedicated team of employees, from the receptionist, to exercise physiologists, to the dietitian, to the psychologist, to nurses and volunteers, we have been able to show almost the same success as Dr. Dean Ornish.

The only difference between our program and the Dean Ornish program is that we allow our patients to eat a little meat. In spite of our sincere efforts by patients and staff it was impossible to get these Midwesterners, who are meat-and potato-eating folks, to be completely vegetarian.

To be fair, it is really difficult to become vegetarian because we are generally taught to cook and eat with meat as the primary ingredient. In 1991 if you went out to eat it was difficult to find food which was completely vegetarian and tasty. Of course now there are a lot of new businesses coming up that serve a nice vegetarian dinner, particularly on the West Coast. Most of our patients who have shown the reversal of heart disease by lifestyle changes consume fifteen to seventeen percent of their calories from fat. Hardworking staff members and patients who believed in the program and I have shown that the reversal of coronary artery disease is not just a dream but can be done by anyone who is willing to make the necessary changes to have a healthy heart. People who are successful in reversing the disease have made substantial changes in their lives to achieve that success.

I am not saying that our program to prevent or reverse coronary artery disease through a low fat diet, exercise, and stress management is the only way a person can prevent or reverse heart disease, but it is *one* way that I know which works. People are not born with heart disease; it is a disease of Western culture. Wherever the abundance of food has occurred, cardiac disease has increased. This observation has been supported by numerous international studies.

When I looked at myself, with no family history of coronary artery disease, no high blood pressure, no diabetes, a cholesterol level under 220, and a lifelong nonsmoker, I started wondering why I had this disease. I reached the conclusion that bad management of stress and isolation was the cause of my problem.

In addition, during my stay at Emory Hospital in Atlanta, doctors revealed to me that I had a little-known gene abnormality, LP(a), in my blood. A lipoprotein particle, LP(a), a genetic variation of LDL cholesterol, has been identified in patients with premature heart disease. Quite a few scientific papers have been written on this subject, but the role of LP(a) is still unclear, and not enough is known to make a definitive statement. I have collected data from studies involving my own patients also and have found the Lp(a) to be very important risk factor in the process of atherosclerosis. I am convinced that if you have a high level of Lp(a), a low level of HDL, and high blood sugar, then your chances of premature heart disease is high. The only treatment for this is a high dose of niacin; however, the problem is that it is not easy to take such a high dose of niacin. Problems include itching, dry skin and flushing, and in my practice more than seventy percent of the patients could not take niacin at dosage levels that could help lower the LP(a) to the desired range.

The other thing touted these days is the *homosystine* blood level. Unfortunately this is a very costly test to perform, but the treatment is very cheap—taking a vitamin known as folic acid. It may cost only about four dollars a month, there are practically no side effects, and it is available without prescription.

I believe that stress management is an extremely important factor in causing heart disease and an important factor in preventing and or reversing heart disease. My research indicates that 67 percent of the patients I have seen in the rehabilitation center are not there because of high cholesterol, but rather due to an abnormal stress profile. Before talking with each patient about a plan of action, I look over the patient's entire psychological profile first to see if the person is resistant to change, is hostile, and/or is impulsive. If these traits are part of a person's psychological makeup, I know that it will be difficult for the patient to accept the lifestyle changes needed to prevent a coronary artery disease or stop the progression or reversal of the heart disease. If I cannot change a person's psychological behavior, then I am wasting his or her time telling him or her what to eat and how to exercise. The psychological factor has become the focus and foundation of this program. Patients must convince themselves that it is only they who have a control of their lives and can change the problem. As I advise my patients, "It is your body, and if you don't take care of it nobody else will, either. You have to have a mission to want to change your lifestyle. Are you doing all of this for you, or are you doing it for your kids? You have to do it for *yourself.*"

The good Lord knows when our time is coming on our one-way ticket through this universe. I am not going to spend the last few years of my life in a nursing home if I can do anything to prevent that. I would like to go the same day the good Lord is ready to take me and definitely not prolong my life with artificial machines and other modern medical marvels. If you want to see the Taj Mahal of modern medicine, visit the coronary care units in a hospital. You will realize how much medicine has advanced in the last twenty-five years.

Personally, I am not interested in the quantity of life—the number of years we live. I am interested in the quality of life. I can live the good life only if I make it happen, doing things such as exercising regularly, eating the right kind of food, and making stress work for me through positive thoughts, just as the little girl taught me to do.

Health care has the potential to bankrupt our country. I believe that if people understand and act, they can change the system. Politicians and insurance companies are not going to do anything to change the system. This country was made by the people and for the people. We have the power to change, but we can change our country's health only if we understand that *we* need to change ourselves first. Only then can we work to change others.

I always tell my patients when they graduate from the program that they must go out and persuade two more people to change their lifestyle so that we can protect our health care system from going broke. My graduates must act as "points of lights." It is incumbent on them to share their knowledge with their family and teach their kids how to live in this environment and strengthen their three pillars of life. I tell them, "You must share with them how you have learned to create a healthy heart and convince them that if you can do it, then why don't they?"

I have taken some of my philosophy from other physicians, like Dr. Robert Eliot, author of the book, *Is It Worth Dying For?* and Dr. Bernie Siegel, author of many books on health and healing. All of these philosophies, along with mine, have been built into our cardiac rehabilitation program. These philosophies not only have helped patients to stop the progression of their heart disease but also to reverse it.

Live in the present moment.
Exercise because you must.
Eat for your health and not for your body.
Stress can be a virtue, but don't make it a killer.

4

Cardiac Prevention and Reversal

"When you were born, you cried and everybody rejoiced. Live such a life that when you die everybody cries and you rejoice."—Anonymous

IN THE PAST TWENTY YEARS THE FIELD OF CAR-diology has made tremendous progress towards saving the heart muscle. This marvel has been achieved by using newer medications, newer clot busters, angioplasty and bypass surgery.

The heart is actually a pump whose sole purpose is to circulate the blood in the body. With a big thump repeated about seventy times a minute, blood is pumped by the heart through the arterial highways of the body. Then through the small arteries, the streets, blood is finally delivered to the small cells, delivering the most important nutrient for the body called oxygen in an act of precision. For in exactly the same amount of time, the blood gushes back with a thump, like a sudden vacuum action, to bring all the blood back to the heart through the back roads called veins.

Whenever you are diagnosed to have a heart disease from stress testing or cardiac catheterization, or after you have had a heart attack, you may be offered either of the two forms of medical advice. Depending on the comfort level of your physician you will either be referred to an invasive cardiologist, who specializes in using different tools to do angioplasty, which is supposed to open up the blocked artery, or to a cardiothoracic surgeon, who specializes in doing open-heart surgery.

Statisticians tell us that the death rate from heart disease in our nation has dropped by about 45 percent since the early 1970s. That seems encouraging. We, the physicians who have been practicing the Western style of medicine definitely are making an impact on this disease. That is why we have been able to drop the *death rate*! Notice, I said the *death rate*. I did not say the *incidence* of heart disease. Heart disease is still the Number One Killer in the USA. Every year 600,000 people die of this preventable disease. *Every Minute one person* is dying of this preventable disease in our country.

Nobody is denying that the newer medical and surgical advances played a major role in decreasing this commendable drop in death rate. These include new medications such as clot busters and the electronic Taj Mahal of medical gadgets in our hospitals, and those brave paramedics in their ambulances including the ACLS (Advanced Cardiac Life Support) trained emergency medical staff in the hospitals. But all of this success has been achieved at a substantial price. We have started asking, "Can we afford all of this?" "Can we spend our scarce medical dollars for a disease which is completely preventable?"

You and I know that is too costly to get sick anymore. If you can afford to see the doctor I hope you have prescription insurance to cover the cost of the medications. It is disturbing that sometime you may have to choose between food and medicine. This is true in the heartland. I have seen that during my active practice. I used to ask those wonderful medical reps to give me as many drug samples as they could so that I could share them with my needy patients. Is this the price we are ready to pay for our health and for the diseases which are preventable? I don't believe so. With those two alternatives presented to you after being diagnosed with heart diseases—angioplasty and/or bypass surgery—let me present to you a **third** alternative: reversal of heart disease by life style changes. I feel that focusing on the power of prayer, the mind and body connection, the power of self realization and awareness, being responsible for your own body, getting rid of isolation, ego and stress, using meditation and prayer for self healing represent the other way of managing your heart disease.

Two out of three patients that I have seen in our cardiac rehabilitation program are there because of the toxic stress. By toxic stress I mean that they have problems being impulsive, egoistic, anger prone, hostile and depressed. Almost all of them are resistant to change. Stress itself is not a problem, but how we handle stress may be. It is not the perception of an event, but the way we react to the event that becomes the problem.

I always say that heart disease is like a mosaic. Those beautiful, bright stained glass pieces carefully put together to make a picture are called a mosaic. There is no single cause of heart disease. Like a mosaic, it is a disease of many factors. You don't get heart disease if you only have a high cholesterol level or if you only have high blood pressure. You get this disease when you have been successful in putting together all the pieces which make up the heart disease mosaic.

Basic ways of preventing heart disease are not to start smoking or to quit smoking, lower your intake of dietary fat and cholesterol, exercise regularly, practice stress management techniques, and keep an ideal body weight. Following these guidelines will be your best defense against heart disease.

What I just said sounds easy but is it really ? Of course not. Otherwise why would you be reading this book?

It has been scientifically established that any individual can influence the course of heart disease through lifestyle changes. The aforementioned guidelines are key factors in preventing and reversing heart disease. People who have a strong genetic predisposition to heart disease can improve their risk profile through the use of appropriate drugs and lifestyle changes. Many people who experience abnormal lipids can improve their health without drugs by practicing lifestyle changes in diet, exercise, and stress management.

Dean Ornish, MD, had the vision and mission to treat this ravage of heart disease by treating the cause of the disease rather then the symptoms. Although not taken seriously initially, later on his findings gained respect in the medical community. Even then everybody was skeptical about how successful one could be in making the American public at large become a vegetarian, taking only ten percent of calories from fat. I personally think that Dr. Ornish will be respected in the medical literature as the first to present an alternative course of medicine to treat heart disease. As a pure researcher he did show what he believed in: that a change of lifestyle can cause the reversal of the disease. Publishing the data in important medical journals, he was able to show that with aggressive lifestyle changes which included one hour of meditation everyday, a vegetarian diet using ten percent of calories from fat, (normal consumption of American diet fat is forty percent) and three hours of aerobic exercise every week, one can stop the progression and initiate reversal of heart disease.

About at the same time Dr. Schuller from Germany showed that he could produce almost the same results by letting his patients exercise in a group for 30 minutes a day. He recommended a stress management program and put the patients on a diet regimen which allowed only twenty percent of calories from fat. Then the FATS study done by Greg Brown from Seattle, Washington, showed that you could attain almost the same results by putting the patients on an

American Heart Association Diet of thirty percent calories from fat diet with exercise and cholesterol-lowering medications. Although the "gold standard" was the Ornish program, people started trying different programs to see the different results.

When I began a cardiac rehabilitation program. I started aggressively using Dean Ornish philosophy and program. Soon, however, I realized that this was not going to work here. I was trying to implant the program from the West Coast to a small town in the Midwest which, needless to say, is a meat-and-potato country where people raise farm animals for a living. After about six months, I decided to modify his program to suit my community. I took a middle road approach and came up with a reasonable plan that my patients were ready to accept.

That is how the "Modified Reversal Program" came in to existence in my practice in 1991. My program was simple. If you don't want to be "sad," **S.A.D.**, then follow this improved program:

    S. Stress management   Smoking
    A. Aerobic exercise   Alcohol
    D. Diet   Drugs

In brief, this is how this program works. Every item will be discussed in detail in following chapters.

Stress and stress management

Can stress be the cause of heart disease?

The answer to that is a resounding YES. Two out of three of our patients are in rehab because of some kind of stress and the problem of coping with related illness. Notice, I am saying "stress" and "coping with related illness." Since 1953 when the term "stress" was coined, it has been literally abused to death. Just to define what stress means will give you stress. All of us, myself included, abuse this term so much that we really don't know what stress actually means. It is not the word "stress" that causes the problem. How you handle it is the key. Coping properly is where we need to work. To help you learn to cope you must understand what stress really means to you in your situation. Lifestyle changes can be achieved only if you understand what else has been going on in your life.

Before I see a patient I always evaluate his or her computerized psychological profile report, which is provided to us in questionnaire form by the patients themselves. This is the most important piece of information for me to help patients in the difficult task of changing their lifestyle. The coping problems I look for are:

Resistance to change, impulsive nature, hostility, Type A personality, depression

If a patient is resistant to change and is very impulsive, I will be wasting his time if I can't convince him or her what part of his personality has not let him change in spite of his efforts in the past.

If the patient is type A and has hostility along with that, then this becomes a toxic stress. For this patient my approach would be different. All this will be discussed in the chapter on stress management.

I also found that meditation using mantras and other fancy stuff, although accepted in the West, was not accepted here. So with the help of a very well trained yoga teacher we offered meditation courses using Dr. Benson's technique of saying ONE rather than anything else. For more on this topic, see Chapter 7, which deals with stress and stress management.

Smoking

I have one piece of advice for everybody: **STOP SMOKING!**. For any macho men who still are not listening, my usual advice is that smoking is the number one cause of impotency. To stop smoking is the single, most powerful change you could undertake to alter the course of heart disease.

Aerobic Exercise

My recommendation is to exercise aerobically in the prescribed aerobic heart rate (See page 117) for one hour every other day or thirty minutes a day, using most of the lower body muscles on a treadmill, rower and bicycle. Seventy percent of muscle is found in the lower part of the body; the chest wall muscles biceps and shoulders make up only about thirty percent. To burn fat you need muscle, so it is important to train and prep your fat-burning muscles first so that they can do a good job helping you to burn that ugly fat

Alcohol

My advice to my patients is not to drink more than two drinks a day for men and not more then one drink a day for women. And you are *not* allowed to accumulate the total for the weekends! Drinks should be sipped and enjoyed slowly. Alcohol is absorbed into the blood stream quickly and taken to the liver for detoxification so that it is fit for consumption by the body. Alcohol actually is a toxin and for the liver to detoxify it properly it has to be delivered slowly; a sudden gush of alcohol can cause toxic effects. This is advice, not a prescription. If you are not drinking, don't make an effort to start now. There are conflicting reports of the positive effects of alcohol on your heart.

Diet

I recommend limiting fat intake in the diet to about 15 to 17 percent of total calories from fat. I have allowed my patients to consume fish, white meat of turkey and skinless chicken breast. If people want to eat beef we allowed them to eat a piece equal to the size of the deck of cards once a week. Although meat eating is permitted in my program, I encourage my patients to eat more fruit, vegetables, nuts, soybean and other vegetarian products.

Drugs

I am extremely aggressive with my patients about treating their abnormal cholesterol particularly good (HDL cholesterol) and Bad (LDL cholesterol), adjusting them to the expected levels.

In early 1992 I was pleased when our first star patient was studied by cardiac catheterization to check his reversal of heart disease. As we were hoping, he did reverse his coronary artery disease. We also tried to show reversal in different patients using different investigative techniques because it was costly to put every patient through the cardiac catheterization. We tried the thallium technique using the same camera and the same technician to avoid mechanical or technical mistakes. We correlated patients' improvement on the VO_2 stress testing and also looked into the increase in MET level.

VO_2 stress testing measures heart and lung endurance, the most important component of physical fitness. Progressive treadmill exercises measure the maximum capacity of oxygen that can be delivered from the air to the body's tissues. The higher the VO_2 rating, the more efficient the body is in oxygenizing the tissues, and the better aerobic capacity and fitness of the person being tested.

MET (Metabolism Equivalent Testing) is a medical term we use to express the metabolic equivalent of physical activity, the rate of energy expended by the human body to achieve aerobic capacity.

I am comfortable now checking my patients' recovery using non invasive measurements. I give most of the credit of reversal to the patients themselves. This is not an easy thing to do. Who wants to get out of bed early in the morning to exercise? Who want to skip that tray of mouth-watering doughnuts? Only those who have commitment, vision or mission to achieve their goal to have and create a healthy heart can succeed. That is the commitment I am encouraging you to make. I did it. Why don't you?

My feeling is that you can not achieve the goal unless you are properly prepared to do so. To reverse heart disease, the vision or mission is vital. You need to be educated about what is the cause of your heart disease, why it happened to you, and what can you do now to reduce chances for further damage. You must accept one fact: you are lucky to be alive. Out of 1.2 million people who are stuck with this disease, only half of you survive. If you have suffered from coronary artery disease, you must realize that you have been lucky to get another chance. I thank the good Lord for your good fortune and urge you to commit yourself to creating a healthy heart for yourself and for your family and friends.

Have you ever asked yourself why you got heart disease? The answer is usually easy. It is your lifestyle. There are three things we have no control of. One is genetics, one is geriatrics (aging) and the third is gender. We all know that men have more chance of heart disease before the age of fifty then women do, although this observation is changing pretty fast as more and more women are subjected to stresses of the work force. The incidence of heart disease among women is increasing, too. Women enjoy lower rates of heart disease until about age fifty, but within seven to ten years after that they catch up with men.

Today women may hold three jobs: working at the office, taking care of home and kids and taking care of their husbands. (The third one may be the biggest challenge of all). All of this work makes more and more of women come to us with early heart disease. When I started in 1991 only 38 percent of our population in the Cardiac Rehabilitation Center were women; in 1996, 46 percent of them were women. The average age of women in the cardiac rehabilitation unit has dropped by about six years. This phenomenon is reported nationally.

Even worse is the fact that more and more *kids* are coming to the cardiac rehab program. I call them "kids" because they are so young. I am talking about people who are in their early thirties. I am afraid that we are going to see more and more of them if we don't change the trend of teenage smoking and life in the fast lane.

My prevention and reversal plan is based on your heart-to-heart commitment to fight heart disease. This is a life-long commitment made with dedication and determination. Some people require only subtle lifestyle changes while others must totally change their way of living. You must put forth serious effort, sacrifice as needed to improve the quality of your life and lower your chances of heart disease.

I am going to outline a plan for you for the prevention and reversal of heart disease. I am committed to help you achieve your goals. I do not believe that healing is a coincidence. People who make miraculous recoveries have invariably made important, positive changes toward a more healthy lifestyle. Don't forget that I, too, had heart disease, and that I have reversed it. Therefore, I can help you to prevent or reverse your heart disease.

Filling out the following data sheet will help you determine appropriate levels and measurements so that you can make objective decisions about what you will do to give your heart a better chance at good health.

Personal Data for Prevention and Reversal of Coronary Artery Disease

1. Cholesterol level: _____mg/dl.
Should be less than 180.

2. HDL Cholesterol: _____mg/dl.
Should be more than 45.

3. LDL Cholesterol: _____mg/dl.
Should be less than 90.

4. LPa (Lipoprotein Alpha): _____mg/dl.
Should be less than 30.

5. Triglyceride level: _____mg/dl.
Should be less than 200.

6. Blood sugar (glucose): _____mg/dl.
Should be less than 110.

7. Blood pressure: _____
A good reading is 120/80.

8. Body weight: _____
Should be within 5% of normal limits.

9. Exercise (aerobic): _____
Should be 30 minutes a day

10. Stress: _____
Should be managed well

11. Diet: _____
Should be balanced, low-fat

12. Smoking: _____
Zero. Stop it or don't start.

5

Patients in the Program

"For a man to conquer himself is the first and noblest of all victories."—Plato (428-348 BC)

DOES THE PROGRAM WORK? WHEN I SAY, "I did it, why don't you?" perhaps I should say, "If *we* could do it so could you." I would like you to read for yourself about a few patients whose lives were turned around by my modified Reversal of Heart Disease program.

What unites all of our patients is an overwhelming desire to take control of their lives. They are all committed to better health through a balanced, low fat diet, exercise, and stress management. A thread of gratefulness runs through all of them—gratitude for a second chance in life. They all express a strong personal faith and a sense of peace in their lives. In addition, they have strong family or friendship bonds. These patients are convinced of their own role in achieving good health, and they do not take life for granted.

Lastly, they are convinced that the mind plays a role in the body's healing process.

Changes are never easy. You need a personal commitment to make this type of change and set a precise goal for really wanting to change. Without a clear mission to change, you will not be blessed with long-lasting pleasure in attaining your goal. Some people want to lose weight but only for the outward appearance and pleasure. Once that goal is met, they are happy for a little while, then reverse to the old habits because the goal was met and the happiness was short lived. The same is true for making lifestyle changes to protect your heart. I often have heard patients say that they wanted to lose pounds to fit in a specific dress for a marriage, or some other special occasion, but then what? Once you achieve that short-term goal, your mind will not support you any more because that is all you have trained your mind to achieve. Once the goal is met, that's it; You lose incentive because your defined goal has been achieved.

It's your mind you need to work on. You need to convince it that you really do want to get your lazy body to exercise every day, to eat healthy low-fat food, and change your high-drive personality. You are changing it to improve your intrinsic quality of life and don't want to be SAD any more then you could gain long-lasting happiness.

When I got sick the first time I did not pay much attention to my mind and body. I was thinking that since I had bypass surgery, I would be good for at least ten years and only in the last couple of years would I have to be more careful. But when I learned that almost all the bypass grafts had closed in about a year and when I almost died on the table while having my angioplasty an year later, that got my attention. I was scared.

One thing I can say is that I am not afraid of death anymore. I know that when my time comes nobody can stop that, even in the best hospital in the world. I believe that for each of us our time frame is already defined in this one-way ticket journey. Once we can accept that as a fact we can decide for ourselves what we really want from life?

Do we want a good quality of life or we rather take it as it comes with no thoughts to consequences? After my angioplasty I chose to change my lifestyle for two reasons. One is that I felt connected with the good Lord, and I relinquished control over my life. The other reason was that I wanted to live a quality life while I had it. I wanted to be happy and nondependent until death comes. I realized that only I can shape my future. I was apprehensive about having a stroke and prolonging my life in a nursing home. I did not want to take a detour of my life through a nursing home.

You may want to ask me why, if I trust the Lord so much, do I think I can change the future? Hey! My answer to that is very simple: the only thing I said was that the good Lord is the only one who knows when that one-way ticket expires. This does not mean that you should abuse your body and the privilege of life. To maintain this marvelous God-given gift, you must take charge and play an important role in keeping your body healthy. Stress management. aerobic exercise and eating right are the methods to achieve it.

After my second incident I felt as if somebody had hit me with a two-by-four. I woke up and seriously started examining where I had gone wrong. It did not take me long to figure out that unmanageable stress was one of the problems. The next step was figuring out how to handle this problem. Once affected by the coronary artery disease a person actually has a 100 percent chance of having a stroke also. Knowing this was enough to scare me into changing my lifestyle and taking control of my risk factors.

Let me tell you why I am so scared of a stroke. This story begins with a patient of mine that I used to take care of when I was actively practicing. I still remember Martha, my patient, who was in her seventies, a beautiful woman with high blood pressure. Her husband had died a few years earlier and she was still missing him. I suspect this was the cause of her high blood pressure. She was always beautifully dressed. Her clothes were always neat and her hair nicely permed. Her shoes always matched her clothes. I would say that she was the most neatly dressed woman I had ever seen. However, she would never exercise, and she would cook only TV dinners. I used to ask her to exercise and take care of herself. She would gently smile and acknowledge my suggestions, but would never listen to me. I was afraid of her having a crippling disease, particularly a stroke. She had no family member living close and I knew if something happened to her, she would have go to a nursing home. It would be difficult for me to see her that way.

Sure enough, one day I got a call from the hospital that she was in the emergency room with a stroke. One side of her body was not functional (hemiplegia), and she was unable to speak, which meant that she was aphasic. I quickly reached the hospital and started her on all those medications available to decrease the pressure in the brain, hoping that I could at least be able to save her speech. A neurologist friend of mine tried to help also, but she was completely paralyzed. The damage was already done. She had been in this state for two days lying on her kitchen floor before a neighbor found her and called the ambulance. If she had been attended to promptly we could have prevented at least part of the damage.

(That is why I always tell my patients that if they have an abnormal chest pain, please go immediately to the emergency room to get it checked. It is always better to be safe than sorry. Never be ashamed of going to the hospital and worrying if everything is OK people will think you are a hypochondriac. Believe me, we would be much happier to see you early and healthy rather than when you are having a full-blown heart attack.)

After a few days in the hospital Martha had to be transferred to the nursing home. There was no other alternative. My wife suggested that we should bring her home, but there was really no choice but to send her to the nursing home for round-the-clock medical care. I visited her once a month and had mixed feelings about her. I was angry at her because she hadn't listened to me, but at the same time I felt sorry for her when I used to see her sitting in the chair in the hallway of the nursing home, slumped to one side, her face drawn and drooling saliva from the angle of her mouth with saliva all over her clothes and the supporting table. Her hair was always messed up and never in place as it used to be. She would be wearing a hospital gown with the slit in the back and brown hospital socks. She was a prisoner in her own body. So many times I would go home with tears in my eyes.

Because the nursing home nurses and aids knew about my feelings, they would always take extra time to dress her up before I came to see her. I would sit in front of her asking questions about her with the nurse standing next to me but she never spoke back to me. She would just stare at me. Once in a while she would mumble a few words but most of the time the visit was one-sided. She died peacefully one night with no heroic measures taken. I have no idea what was on her mind when she would stare at me, what she was trying to tell me. I still can't forget those eyes. This incident changed me. It gave me a strong reason to do my best to avoid having a stroke or a crippling disease which may incapacitate me in this way. I will do my best so that when my time comes I may be able to die on my terms. To achieve this goal of having a good quality of life, I had to take charge of my life and work. The Lord helps those who help themselves.

My mission began when I decided to change my lifestyle and my determination to share this vision with my kids, wife and friends followed. To share both my mission and my vision I started the Coronary Prevention and Rehabilitation Program, which would help me and my patients. To sincerely convey my mission I practiced what I preached. I am sure this is one of the main reasons why this program is so successful. The mission message was literally coming from my heart. Because I myself had heart bypass surgery and angioplasty, my patients believed what I had to tell them. People listen to those to whom they feel bonded by the same experience. They know that I have been in their shoes. They know this advice is not coming from a textbook but from my heart. Their trust in me has helped them to gain confidence in my mission and vision to change and to take control of their lives.

Let me share with you some of my exemplary patients, my "points of light," who have been able to make those changes in themselves and helped their families and friends in accepting a healthy lifestyle. I will also share with you techniques by which to judge each of their achievements.

Patient # 1

Charles Beard, 67 years old, a retired community college professor, a former Type A personality with no family history of heart disease. Charles had a heart attack at the age of 62 which resulted in slight damage to the heart muscle. Bypass surgery followed, with two bypass grafts done at this time.

After surgery he did everything he was advised to do, but two years later he had chest pain, which caused him to go to the hospital. There he was subjected to another angiogram, which revealed that one of his bypass grafts was closed. The original artery, which was bypassed in the first surgery, was still 98 percent closed. The bypass on this artery had failed. He was advised to undergo an angioplasty of that artery or have another bypass surgery, which he opted to defer until he could find out the real cause of early closure of the bypass. He did not understand why the bypass had failed in just two years.

When Chuck read about Dr. Dean Ornish's program he decided to join our Reversal Program. Initially I was a little reluctant to have him in the program because he had begun to have frequent angina pain with a little exertion. Nevertheless, seeing his dedication, I accepted him in the program.

A previous cigarette smoker and occasional pipe smoker for fifteen years, Chuck had stopped smoking at the age of thirty-five. Throughout his teaching career, Chuck had always felt a certain amount of stress. He had a toxic stress personality (a Type A personality with hostility). His HDL (good cholesterol) was low. This is, of course, a deadly combination. Six out ten patients who are in the Cardiac Rehabilitation program have this combination. I can't prove it, but I believe this combination of factors has something to do with abnormal cortisol release. Patients who have toxic stress usually release too much adrenaline and cortisol. This in turn affects the liver, causing either low release of HDL or excessive utilization of HDL by the body causing a decrease in the HDL pool.

Outgoing and optimistic, Chuck and his wife became true vegetarians to improve the quality of their lives. Chuck was aware of the Dean Ornish Diet, and he and his wife accepted the modified program with enthusiasm. Their daily intake of fat remains under 30 grams. Through a major change in diet and exercise, Chuck has maintained a 28-pound weight loss. He and his wife enjoy a glass of wine with dinner and are conscientious about their food selections.

Encouragement from his wife and others exerted a positive influence on Chuck's attitude. This helped him to make the necessary changes in diet, exercise, and stress reduction to reverse his coronary artery disease. Over time, his exercise capacity has increased tremendously. He can now do more than he has ever been able to do in the past. His chest pain has almost gone now, and stress tests have shown remarkable improvement.

Golfing and yard work in the summer, in addition to three one-hour weekly sessions throughout the year at the Rehab Center keep Chuck physically active. He also exercises on equipment at his home.

By interacting with others, walking, deep breathing, or utilizing a self- talk technique recommended by Dr. Robert Eliot, author of *Is it worth Dying for?* Chuck has been able to relieve stress.

His belief that one must pick up and go on with one's life indicates that a fulfilling life awaits those who are able to take control of their lives and reverse their coronary artery disease.

The following graph represents one of the ways we monitored progress and that is by calculating the MET'S level (a measurement of metabolic activity, explained on page 190).

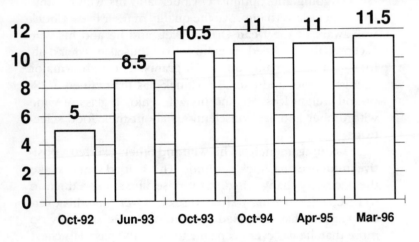

Metabolism Improvement from Exercise (measured in METS)

Patient # 2

Edward Allen, 78, did not discover that he had heart problems until his 74th birthday. At his wife's urging, Eddie had a thorough physical examination which revealed an abnormality on his EKG. Further testing by angiogram indicated a silent heart attack a few years prior to that time and that he had severe blockage of his coronary arteries. Having grown up in various Catholic orphanages, Eddie had no knowledge of his family's medical history.

Eddie's first reaction was disbelief and a desire not to tell anyone the results of his testing. Although he smoked two packs of cigarettes daily for thirteen years as a young man, he had quit cold turkey at the age of thirty-one. Eddie did not correlate his heart disease with his former smoking habit.

A moderate exerciser throughout his life, as a young man he had lifted weights and boxed, and in later years, he swam and cycled. However, thirty-five years as a lithographic pressman, a stressful job that necessitated heavy lifting, had taken its toll.

Eddie, like the majority of Americans, had not been particularly careful in his choice of foods throughout his life. A desire for certain foods dictated his selection without much concern about dietary fats and cholesterol.

Not one to admit defeat, Eddie accepted his coronary artery disease as a blessing in disguise. He has been able to improve his quality of life and lower his cholesterol through major dietary changes, exercise; and stress management. Eddie believes that it is essential to have a positive frame of mind and good self-esteem to make positive changes in one's life.

Eddie has limited his intake of eggs to four soft-boiled eggs per month. He eats lots of pasta, fruits, and vegetables, and small portions of chicken and fish a couple of times a week. He eats lean beef once or twice a month. He gives his full attention to his exercise routine of three weekly one and one-half hour sessions at the Rehabilitation Center.

In addition, he has been successful in reducing stress by playing the organ, reading the Bible, concentrating on his hobby of photography, working at the computer, and listening to music.

Eddie's deep faith, determination, and will power have allowed him to make the necessary changes to improve the quality of his life at an age when others might refuse to try to change old habits. Eddie is living proof that a positive attitude, faith in God, perseverance, and hard work are the necessary tools to change one's life regardless of one's age.

Unfortunately he had to undergo bypass surgery in 1996. In spite of all the investigation I still can't explain the cause of this obstruction. The only factor that I could think of Eddie's experience years earlier while doing a home improvement project. His right hand and arm were exposed to glass fiber insulation while working without any gloves and or proper protective gear. The next day his hand was swollen and painful and continued to be like that for about four or five months. He was in a quite a lot of pain and had several sleepless nights. He developed contractures of his right hand and was in a way crippled with the pain. After a while he was able to exercise a little bit until he was almost back to his former level of fitness.

On his annual stress test he was not able to perform as well as before, although the stress test results were acceptable for his age. He did not have chest pain or any other complaints, but as a precaution a cardiac catheterization was ordered. This test showed a new obstruction, and heart surgery was recommended. He is doing better now and is exercising again. Although I don't have any way to prove it, I suspect that his problem had something to do with the stress that he experienced after his painful and crippling exposure to fiberglass.

I wanted to share this patient with you because in spite of all the success we have been able to achieve, we still have so much to learn. This fact usually keeps our life in perspective. Here, in such a case one realizes that in spite of medical marvels and progress we have been able to make we should never let our egos run away with us, never try to compete with the good Lord.

Patient # 3

Having retired from a stressful career as a high school math teacher, David Kludy, 58, has taken control of his life and lifestyle to combat a family history of heart disease which included the death of a 34-year-old brother from a heart attack while canoeing.

Dave's own cardiac problems surfaced in May, 1991, after two heart attacks less than a month apart required him to have quadruple bypass surgery and a mitral valve replacement as a result of blockage of the coronary arteries.

Also in April and August of 1992 he had a repeat mitral valve replacement and a single bypass, when the mitral valve tore loose from deteriorated heart muscle tissue.

Prior to the third mitral valve replacement, Dave was scheduled for a heart transplant. As a result of his insurance company's reluctance to pay for the transplant, Dave was sent to the Cleveland Clinic for a second opinion. There doctors performed the third and final mitral valve replacement.

Dave's cardiac problems had resulted from a sedentary lifestyle, an extremely stressful job, and unregulated eating habits. Dave has made major changes in three areas of his life—exercise, diet, and stress management—to improve his cardiac profile.

Dave exercises three times a week at the Coronary Prevention and Rehabilitation Center. In addition, he walks one to two miles three times a week with his wife around a high school track near his home. In spring and summer, he gardens and mows his two and one-half acre yard with a self-propelled lawn mower.

Dave, who eats out twice a week, advises others to order healthy side dishes instead of unhealthy entrees. At fast food restaurants, Dave orders baked potatoes and chooses wisely from the salad bar instead of eating high fat and caloric foods like hamburgers and french fries. Not a vegetarian, Dave opts for turkey instead of red meat, which he rarely eats, and has eliminated all dairy and egg products from his diet.

In the area of stress management, Dave reduced most of his tension and stress upon retirement. His belief that attitude towards one's body directly influences physical health has led him to worry less in his life. His ability to replace worrisome thoughts with good ones has given him peace of mind. When feeling stressed, Dave reads to distract his mind, exercises, or turns to one of his hobbies such as gardening to relax.

Through these changes, Dave has reversed his coronary artery disease, lowered his cholesterol, and learned the contentment that comes from taking control in those areas of life that are controllable.

Dave has a deep belief in God and strong family and friendship bonds which have helped him weather his heart disease. Dave could not change his heredity; therefore he changed his lifestyle and lowered his risk of future, debilitating heart disease.

Patient # 4

A high level of stress, twenty-five years of cigarette smoking, food in the fast lane and little exercise combined to result in a heart attack for a 44-year-old physician friend of mine. Without a family history of heart disease, the physician still found himself faced with heart disease as a result of controllable risk factors, smoking, lack of exercise, and a harder to control factor, stress, in a busy and demanding profession.

One early morning while making rounds in the hospital he began to have chest pain and told a fellow physician that he was not feeling well. In the next couple of minutes his heart stopped, he stopped breathing and was coded right there on the floor. He had a very difficult time in the hospital. He sure is one of the luckiest men alive. If he had coded outside the hospital in the parking lot, I don't think he would have made it. The Lord really had his hand on him.

After a stormy first few days in the Coronary Care Unit he was advised to have an angioplasty which he decide to defer. Instead he joined our reversal program.

This heart attack demanded his attention. The result was that he quit smoking and became a vegetarian with the exception of eating fish. He started exercising aerobically every other day. He also worked hard on stress management. The greatest achievement he made was that he has learned to say *No*. With his dedication to lifestyle changes he was able to reverse coronary artery disease without going through angioplasty.

He believes that everyone needs to become aware of how he or she lives. Awareness is the invitation to change and action is the answer to change. This physician has begun the journey to heal himself in order to live a healthier life.

Following are SPECT Thallium images of his heart before and after the program. Thallium, a nuclear dye, is injected in the patient at the peak of exercise (stress testing) to see the patient's blood supply to the heart when the heart is beating fast. Tagged by the nuclear dye, the blood supply to the heart muscle is monitored by a special camera. In this patient's case, if you look at Picture A and follow the arrows you can see that it looks like someone has taken a bite of the doughnuts. This means that the blood supply to the lower part of the heart has been restricted because of obstruction in the coronary artery. In Picture B, four hours later, the same defect is shown, confirming the diagnosis of an obstructed coronary artery.

After six months in the program, Picture C shows an improvement to the blood supply to the heart muscle during exercise, as does Picture D.

Although the arteriogram remains the "gold standard" to diagnose coronary artery disease, SPECT Thallium and PET Scans are simpler and cheaper alternative ways to follow patients who are participating in a risk reversal program and confirm the reversal of heart disease.

SPECT Thallium Images

A

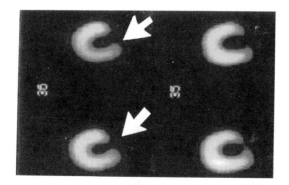

B

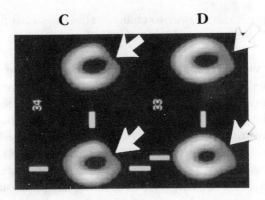

During the resting period of four hours after the stress test, pictures are taken to check the blood supply to the heart at rest. This way we can compare the blood supply to the heart during exercise and at rest. If there is obstruction in the artery, the arteries are not open enough to provide all the tagged blood to the heart muscle. If there is no obstruction the blood supply would be fine. This test to confirm the reversal of heart disease is not only simpler but cheaper.

Patient # 5

Appreciative of what he has in life instead of wishing for what he does not have, Charles Laney, 54, exhibits a positive outlook on life and enjoys it to the fullest. With a family history of heart disease, which includes both parents, Chuck had his first encounter with heart disease in 1982. At age 41 he experienced a heart attack,. Neither a smoker nor drinker, Chuck was not overweight at the time of his heart attack. His cholesterol was high, and he had a high blood pressure also, for which he was being properly treated. In addition to his heart attack, Chuck underwent triple and quadruple bypass surgeries. After the surgery he changed his lifestyle. He was careful about his diet and began an exercise program recommended by his physician.

In January of 1983, Chuck had his first bypass surgery and by the end of the first year his bypass grafts were closed. Chuck continued to watch his diet and kept on exercising until 1989 when he underwent bypass surgery for the second time. By May 1990 his bypass grafts were all closed. Chuck had two angioplasties in 1990 and early 1991, all of which failed after a short period of time.

His cardiologist told him that he might have to undergo heart transplant surgery in the future because of persistent failure of bypass surgery and angioplasties. At the young age of fifty he was determined not to throw in the towel yet.

He joined the reversal program in early 1991 and with his dedication and positive outlook, Chuck has been able to reverse his coronary artery disease through the intensity of his exercise, a completely overhauled vegetarian diet—in which his fat intake is limited to between 10 and 15 grams daily—and a reduction in stress by improving his coping skills.

By exercising one to two hours three to five times weekly, Chuck has been able to decrease the amount of plaque in his coronary arteries and developed collateral circulation around the blockage of the arteries. Carefully watching his diet, he feels comfortable eating out since he knows how to select wisely from the menu.

Being retired, Chuck does not experience the stress he felt when working. Through meditative techniques such as yoga, relaxation exercises and deep breathing, he has learned to control his day-to-day stress.

Chuck believes that the quality of one's life is extremely important. He points out that no one is guaranteed a longer life. However, Chuck believes that people need to take control of their lives and take care of themselves. He states that doctors can tell you *how* to take care of yourself, but you must do it for yourself. Chuck's belief that one should keep a positive attitude and not let anxiety take over one's life reflects the healthy lifestyle and attitudes that he has developed.

He was the first of our patients for whom we were able to document reversal of coronary artery disease. The first picture is of a cardiac catheterization of Chuck's diseased artery of the heart taken in 1991. Follow the arrows. You will see the obstruction of one of his arteries in the first picture. Now notice the angiographic picture of the artery of his heart after one year. By following the arrows you can see that the artery has opened up.

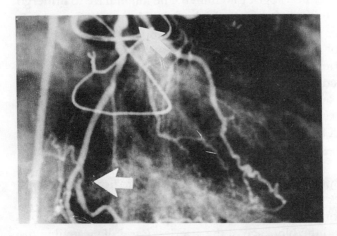

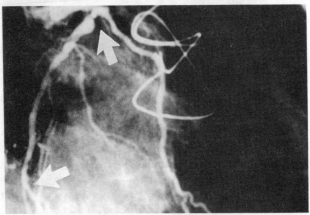

We can never open the arteries to 100 percent of their original capacity. We can only stabilize and shrink the soft plaque. The hard plaque is all calcium, and it is not possible to completely dissolve these calcium deposits. However, by opening up part of the artery and developing a natural bypass around the obstruction, we can be sure that the heart's muscle will receive an ample blood supply, a reversal of the previous situation when blood flow to the heart was restricted.

Chuck was awarded our first "patient of the year" award in 1992. He has been a very active volunteer in our Cardiac Rehab. A mentor to many patients who join the program, he practices what he preaches.

Patient # 6

Mix a Type A personality, a hot temper, lack of exercise, not enough rest, and fifty pounds of excess weight. That recipe describes Donald Fielder, who experienced a heart attack at the age of 52.

Don has undergone a metamorphosis to become healthy. He changed his personality from Type A to Type B. He has learned to control his temper more often than he did before his heart attack. He exercises three times a week at the Rehab Center, and he routinely walks on his treadmill at home. He has given up a lot of activities and has taken himself out of the fast lane and has reduced his weight by 47 pounds, limiting his daily intake to fewer than 10 grams of fat.

Even though Don, with no family history of heart disease, did push-ups and sit-ups daily prior to his heart attack, he believes that stress, his previous eating habits, and lack of cardiovascular exercise all contributed to his heart disease.

By making the above changes, Don has made a successful recovery from his heart attack and single bypass surgery. Recent testing indicates no permanent damage to his heart.

Don believes that people need to remove fat from their diets, lose weight, and practice stress management. When Don feels stressed, he uses a technique known as self-talk to calm himself down and stay in control.

Mix together a sense of control, exercise, healthy eating habits, a calmer life, and the ability to walk away from a stressful situation without exploding and you have a new man: Don Fielder.

Patient # 7

Fred Gluck, age 70, a retired Air Force Colonel, smoked a pipe for forty years, quitting at the age of 61. Having a strong familial history of heart disease, which included both parents and a brother, he also experienced heart problems in the form of a heart attack which resulted from blocked coronary arteries due to plaque buildup.

Fear of a premature death prompted him to change his behavior in terms of diet, exercise, and stress. As he stated, he changed his eating habits for the rest of his life by reducing his daily intake of fat to approximately ten percent of his caloric intake and lost twenty pounds in the process. He believes that eating an unhealthy diet is not worth dying for. Like all the other cardiac rehab patients, he takes vitamins and antioxidants. He takes Vitamins C, E, B, calcium, magnesium, zinc, beta carotene, lecithin, niacin, aspirin, and a beta blocker.

Always moderately active in life, Fred increased the pace of his exercise routine and is even more conscientious about exercising. He uses free weights and exercises six days a week for at least an hour daily. He also walks two miles on a regular basis.

Fred has managed to bring his stress under control, although he admits to having a short fuse occasionally. He practices yoga and deep breathing exercises to relax when he feels stressed.

As a result of his lifestyle changes, he has increased his HDL cholesterol level, decreased his LDL and overall cholesterol levels, and has not experienced any anginal pain in over two years. Enjoying his life, he wants it to be long, healthy, and happy. He refers to this combination as a good quality of life.

With his dedicated lifestyle changes including a low-fat diet, stress management, exercise and weight training, his cholesterol is always under 150, his blood pressure is always like a 20-year-old man, and his pulse rate is always in the low 50s just like an athlete. His total body fat now is about 12 percent, which indicates that he is in excellent shape.

Patient # 8

With no family history of heart disease, at the age of 55 Gene Brackman began to experience chest pain on exertion several times a day. Even though he traveled frequently, he watched his diet, choose poultry and seafood entrees and limited his intake of red meat to three to five times a week. He walked whenever possible, and sometimes up to twenty miles a week. Gene was a pack-a-day cigarette smoker for twenty-one years before quitting at the age of 40.

Tests run by his family physician confirmed a moderately high blood cholesterol but an extremely high sugar level. Gene was told to lose weight and was put on medication for the high sugar. When the chest pain persisted he was referred to a cardiologist for further evaluation. His stress test was positive and the subsequent cardiac catheterization in May showed an obstructive coronary artery disease, which was causing that chest pain. Angioplasty was performed in September. By this time he had lost 45 pounds, and his blood sugar was normal. Within the next three months the pain reappeared requiring him to undergo two repeat angioplasties because of early closure. After each angioplasty, he was given a 30-second piece of advice to exercise, eat a low-fat diet and to reduce stress.

In 1994, after he started having chest pains again and the doctor suggested another angioplasty, he began to ask if there was a better way to handle this problem. Gene contacted me for consultation after attending one of my lectures at his local church. After the initial visit I made him aware that stress along with lack of proper exercise and diet were the main cause of his disease. I made arrangements for him to take yoga classes and drop all meat, poultry and seafood from his diet. Because he had to fly frequently he decided that he would stay only in hotels with exercise facilities and chose to eat only healthy food.

Initially he had chest pain with a little exercise, but this gradually lessened. In order to combat the angina, Gene made several changes in his lifestyle. He became a vegetarian. He is highly aware of the amount of sugar he consumes and restricts his daily caloric intake to 2200 calories. In addition, Gene significantly increased his daily exercise to a maximum of two hours. On a daily basis, he walks on a treadmill, jogs, and rides a stationary bike. On weekends, weather permitting, he walks from three to five miles per day. Like others in the program, he started taking vitamins and antioxidants and also takes a baby-sized aspirin every day.

Gene now views stress as one small part of his life and concentrates on other more important aspects. When he feels stressed, Gene does deep breathing exercises or yoga to relax himself. Gene is happy to be alive and knows that each day brings new possibilities.

After about one year or so of dedicated lifestyle changes, his recent PET Scan test showed a completely normal and viable heart muscle. Like SPECT Thallium, PET Scan is a study of blood supply to the heart muscle using nuclear tags. The PET Scan is considered more accurate than SPECT Thallium, but is not readily available in smaller facilities.

I am proud of what he has been able to achieve on his own without further invasive intervention. This is what I meant by "closing the faucet rather than mopping the floor." By choosing exercise, proper diet and stress management he was able to avoid another angioplasty or bypass surgery.

Patient #9

In 1991, when Gloria, who was 75 at that time, joined the rehabilitation program she was taking fourteen different medications for angina, diabetes, hypertension and gout. Now she is taking only two! What an achievement! Not only is she saving money on medications; she is feeling better, too.

After a careful review of her need for all those medications I found that she was taking medication for reducing water retention. Whenever you take the water pills you always lose potassium; she was prescribed potassium pills. The potassium pill, along with her arthritis medications was upsetting her stomach; and for her stomach pain she was taking Zantac. The water pill was also making her gout and diabetes worse. Because her gout was bothering her, she took sleeping and pain medications. On top of this, she was taking three different heart medications. I felt strongly that if I could slowly get her to exercise and work with her diet and medications, I should be able to cut down the amount of medications that she was taking. The first order of business was to prescribe a sensible diet that she could live on. The dietitian helped her eat smart. I stopped her water pills, which helped me to dispense with her potassium and Zantac. Slowly, in about a year or so, she was taking only five medications.

Now after five years of hard work at the age of 82 she is taking only two medications. She has lost about fifteen pounds, her blood sugar is well controlled with diet, and exercise and her blood pressure is in the acceptable range too. Her angina is practically gone, and I don't think that she has taken any nitroglycerin for a long time.

Gloria has played an active role in changing old habits and attitudes. She has learned a new way of living, and she feels better and seems happier as a result.

Patient # 10

Bonnia Kinsler was 59 years old when in 1993 she was diagnosed with a severe congestive cardiomyopathy. She did not know what that meant, but she knew that she could not walk more than a block without getting short of breath or coughing all the time.

Cardiomyopathy means that the heart, which is a pump, becomes bulky, something like the bulky overflowing biceps muscles some people have. Bulky heart muscles become tired easily. When she joined the Cardiac Rehabilitation Program Bonnie's Ejection Fraction (EF), which measures the pumping action of the heart, was only 19 percent. Her EF was measured by a MUGA Stress Test which is performed by exercising on a bicycle using a special camera like a CAT Scan. This way we know how strong the heart contracts. You need at least a 40 to 50 percent ejection fraction for the heart to be functioning effectively.

Bonnia was advised to exercise and if there was no improvement, a heart transplant was indicated. Scared of having a heart transplant she joined our rehabilitation program to improve her heart function. She changed her lifestyle and worked on the three pillars of life—improving her diet, exercising and managing stress.

The first hope of improvement came in about nine months when her ejection fraction improved to 26 percent. In 1996, with her dedication to a healthy lifestyle and her desire to create a healthy heart, she was able to improve the ejection fraction to 55 percent. Her cardiovascular fitness is actually above normal now. This was done by sheer determination and hard work and by believing in herself that she could do it. She exercised everyday in the center. She was extremely careful about her diet and still consumes only about 20 percent of her calories from fat. She had her bouts with depression and has at times smoked, but she has worked hard to not do things that she was not supposed to.

Her MUGA Scan pictures of her heart are self explanatory. These three MUGA pictures were taken on 1993, 1994, and 1996. In 1993 her heart was visibly enlarged and dilated. In 1994, it has shown some improvement and 1996 the heart looks normal in size and function. It is not as dilated as it was in 1993.

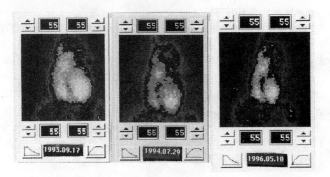

Finally, let me share with you what and how I have been able to achieve and *Create A Healthy Heart* for myself. After my bypass surgery in 1989, the grafts closed within one year. After my near-death experience with angioplasty and its complications in 1991, I was advised to have a second bypass surgery. I chose to refuse this option, accepting instead the alternative way of healing the disease recommended by Dean Ornish. For this I had to make the ultimate sacrifice relinquishing my medical practice that I was trained to provide. It is, of course, not easy to quit what you always have enjoyed doing but for me it was a choice between living and dying.

After my exposure to the Dean Ornish Program I wanted to duplicate the same program in Springfield. Initially, like my patients I started on the Dean Ornish Diet which later on I modified to 15 percent calories from fat. I exercised three times a week for three hours a week in my prescribed aerobic level and started using relaxation and meditation techniques for thirty minutes a day. The relaxation technique is explained in the chapter on stress.

I started an age-old yoga technique, called Surya Namaskar. Before I had heart problems, my dad advised me to do this every day, but I always managed to postpone his advice because I thought I had more important things to do. Surya Namaskar is done every morning after getting out of bed. This is the easiest muscle-relaxing stretching exercise that you can do for your body. (The whole process of Surya Namaskar is explained in the chapter on exercise.) Repeating the procedure five to ten times in the morning will stretch all your muscles. I think this mode of exercise is very important for you to do as you get up in the morning All night your muscles are in a sleeping mode, completely relaxed. But when you get up, the muscles suddenly have to contract to allow your body to perform certain functions. Initially the muscles have to work anaerobically, which produces lactic acid, causing damage to the muscle fiber. Doing this stretching and relaxing exercise daily will help your body muscle to function better all day long. I personally have enjoyed this benefit.

This process of taking control of my health actually made me more connected with myself. I started using more self talk to manage my stress. I began asking myself if a particular situation was worth dying for. My relationship with my kids and wife improved tremendously and I felt better than I had ever felt in my life. And all this was accomplished just by connecting with myself. Learning how to manage stress, I started living in the present moment.

With a regular aerobic exercise regimen, which I do every day with my patients to demonstrate that I practice what I preach, my exercise capacity has improved and my total cardiovascular fitness has improved by about 120 percent. I lost approximately 35 pounds by 1992 and never gained any of them back. This was an extra bonus because I had trained my muscles to burn fat aerobically, so they became efficient fat burning machines. I always say to my patients that when you train your muscles efficiently you will be able to lose your weight and keep it off forever. This is a much better deal than spending so much money on a fancy weight loss program in which statistically 80 percent of them gain the weight back. We actually have a great success with the concept of SAD—Stress management, Aerobic exercise and Diet in our weight loss program—by training muscle to become an efficient fat-burning machine.

I can say from personal experience that prevention or reversal of heart disease involves a very personal commitment of time and energy. For you it will undoubtedly require changing old habits and replacing them with new ones. You will have to change many preconceived ideas about food, exercise, and stress. The program requires a unity of mind, body, and spirit. There is only one person who can make the difference between succeeding or failing—*you*!

6

Women and Heart Disease

There are three words that sweetly blend.
They are "mother," "home" and "Heaven"
—Anonymous

A RECENT UNSCIENTIFIC SURVEY DONE BY ME revealed that the disease that women fear the most is breast cancer. As a matter of fact, most studies echo the same concern among women. A common but dangerous misconception is that women need not worry much about having a heart attack. The facts are that although breast cancer is a big problem, a 50-year-old female is **four to six times** more likely to die from heart disease than breast cancer.

For most of the twentieth century, heart disease has been labeled a man's disease. Until 1993 almost all of the studies on heart disease were focused exclusively on men. In years past, if a woman had chest pains and went to the hospital's emergency room, she was often diagnosed as being nervous or upset and given a tranquilizer. Or, perhaps, she

8 1

was told, the chest tightness was because of pulled muscle, and she was given a muscle relaxant. Or, she might have been told that it was just a case of indigestion, and she was given an antacid to relieve her symptoms. Heart problems also can mirror these or similar symptoms, but doctors simply did not often find heart disease in women.

If a man experienced chest pains and went to the hospital's emergency room, chances are that his complaints were not taken lightly. He would have been immediately put on a heart monitor, an EKG would have been performed, and blood drawn to rule out a heart attack.

The fact is that heart disease is the number one killer of American women, accounting for more deaths than breast, ovarian and cervical cancer **combined.** In 1995, about **40,000** women died of breast cancer while about **500,000** women died of cardiovascular disease. Half of these deaths, **250,000,** are from coronary artery disease but still people, particularly women don't think of heart disease as something that can happen to them.

Women do report to the doctor immediately if they have a lump in their breast or heavy vaginal bleeding, but chest discomfort, nausea or pain is not reported as readily. This neglect of heart symptoms is not women's fault. We in the medical profession have made women believe that this is a man's disease.

In recent years heart disease in women began to receive more attention from the press and the medical community.

The current population of the USA is about 230 million, of whom 118 million, or 51 percent, are women. One-third of these women are 45 years old or older. In 1992 almost seven thousand women died of a heart attack before the age of 40. Women are protected by their hormone, estrogen, up to the age of their menopause. After that they catch up with men pretty quickly and by 60 years of age, the incidence of heart disease in men and women is the same. In 1992, our cardiac rehab center had only 38 percent women with heart disease but now 46 percent of our patients are women. Although I am not happy about reporting this increase in the numbers, it shows the seriousness of the problem.

From the 1960s onward, the majority of women are also breadwinners. Today, women feel the same pressures and stress in the workplace as men do. Besides work stress, women usually go home to another full day's work of cooking, cleaning, and child care. Some things have changed in the 1990s— for example more women are getting help at home from their spouses and children—but the majority working women still bear most of the responsibility for household chores and child care.

Women, like men, now are eating the wrong kinds of food on the run, not getting enough exercise, not getting enough rest, feeling stressed at their jobs and stressed about not being at home for their children, and, like men, too many women are smoking. Is it any surprise, then, that women are also at risk of heart disease?

Let me discuss with you the gender-specific risk factors and what you can do to prevent and or reverse the disease. Smoking, inactivity, diabetes mellitus, hypertension, toxic stress and increased *waist hip ratio* are the major factors that increases the risk of coronary heart disease in women.

Smoking

According to 1993 statistics, 23 percent of women smoke. In 1985, 41 percent of deaths from heart disease in women under the age of 65 resulted from smoking, up from 26 percent in 1965. Women who smoke have a two to six times greater risk of heart disease than women who do not smoke. Women are protected from heart disease till menopause because of the natural hormone estrogen that has an antiatherogenic protective effect, but this effect will be negated by smoking which causes an antiestrogenic effect, which increases platelet clumping and the fibrinogen level. They in turn, cause the blood to clot easily. Cigarette smoking also decreases the HDL cholesterol (good cholesterol) and that may help cause endothelial injury resulting in atherosclerosis.

The national trend of cigarette use by young women aged 20 to 25 years is disappointingly upward, while the rest of society is smoking fewer cigarettes. This trend is very disturbing because this age of woman tends to use contraceptives also. Women who smoke and use oral contraceptives have a very high incidence of heart disease. But remember that although addictive, smoking dependency can be overcome successfully.

Hypertension

Hypertension, or high blood pressure, is twice as common in women with heart disease as in men with heart disease. A rise of only 10 mm Hg (mercury) in diastolic pressure (the bottom number in a blood pressure reading) can increase a woman's risk for heart disease and stroke by 20 to 30 percent.

Diabetes

Diabetes increases the risk of heart disease. Women with diabetes are three times as likely to develop heart disease. Normally a women's coronary artery risk lags about ten years behind men's, but the presence of diabetes abolishes all of this advantage.

Menopause

Heart disease rates increase after natural menopause and peak at about the age of 60. Chronic blood loss in menstruating women may have a preventive effect because of the antioxidant effect of iron depletion. That is why it is thought that aspirin and fish oil may cause chronic blood loss and thus protect women from heart disease. It has been suggested that estrogen replacement therapy (ERT) may be effective in improving a woman's heart risk profile.

Estrogen alone may offer the best protection for women who have no uterus. Natural estrogen may have more cardiac benefits than synthetic estrogen. Hormone therapies do not cause weight gain. However, fewer than one-third of postmenopausal women receive estrogen replacement therapy. Women need to discuss this issue with their physician before starting on this hormonal replacement.

Obesity

A person who is more than 30 percent overweight has a predisposition towards heart disease and stroke. Women who are heavy have a two to three times greater risk of heart attack than do women who are at their ideal weight. The risk is greater for women who carry their extra weight in the abdomen rather than in the buttocks and hips. Gaining weight in adulthood may double the risk, and weight fluctuations are unhealthy. In a large study done by Lapidus and his group in Sweden found that the *waist-to-hip ratio* to be very indicative of coronary risk, particularly if the ratio is more then 0.85. (Divide your waist measurement by your hip measurement for your waist-to-hip ratio.)

Cholesterol

The risk of heart disease is lower when serum cholesterol is below 200 mg/dl. The risk doubles when the level exceeds 240 mg/dl. Apoproteins, the protein component of lipoproteins, may provide a good indicator of heart disease risk, especially apo A-1, a component of HDL; and apo B, the major component of LDL. The higher the ration of apo A-1 to apo B, the lower the risk of heart disease.

A lipoprotein particle, **LPa**, a genetic variation of LDL, has been identified in patients with premature heart disease. With high **LPa** and **low HDL** a diabetic patient indicates a very good chance of having a premature coronary artery disease. A high triglyceride level increased the risk, particularly in women.

Alcohol Intake

Alcohol's role in women's risk for heart disease remains controversial. Some studies have suggested that having a moderate alcohol intake will decrease mortality. I caution all my patients that women should not drink more than one drink a day and definitely should not drink during pregnancy. Because alcohol will increase triglyceride levels, all factors should be considered before running off to the wine store.

Multiple roles

Multiple stressors resulting from greater responsibilities at work and at home increase risk. Some evidence indicates that women who work outside the home may lessen their risk if they become more conscious of appearance, resulting in eating better and exercising.

Stress

The one main risk factor that binds men and women together is toxic stress, known as Type H. Almost seven out of ten patients with coronary artery disease have toxic stress. (For more information on toxic stress, see Chapter 8.)

The rate of heart disease among younger females has increased over the last two decades, perhaps because physicians have become more aware of heart disease in women and are detecting it at an earlier age, and also because more women are smoking. The number of older patients with heart disease also is increasing.

In addition, the rate of recurrence of coronary artery disease in women is higher than that of men. Of 21 women with coronary artery disease whom I followed in a five-year study, four had recurrence of coronary artery disease, one had bypass surgery, two died, and the rest were not following the lifestyle changes recommended to them.

Women are under more stress than ever. Self-care is often neglected. Men do not support women as much as women support men. In our cardiac rehabilitation program, which has been in operation for five years before this book was written, I have noticed that husbands usually do not come to the support group meetings with their wives when the wife is sick; maybe they are working. When the husband is sick, the wife usually is present at almost all of the meetings, lending her moral and psychological support. On average, 75 percent of the wives come with their husbands to these support group meetings, while only 25 percent of the husbands come with their wives. Women, in general, do not receive the same emotional support from their husbands. This lack of emotional support is a most likely cause of repeat coronary artery disease in women.

Clerical workers, especially those who have "blue collar" working husbands and several children, appear to have higher risk of heart disease. The most important predictors are—

A suppressed hostility

A non-supportive boss

Little control over the work environment

Perception of losing control

What can women do to help themselves? Some males are more responsive to the needs of their wives spouses compared with those of ten to twenty years ago. Men and women need to communicate their needs to each other and begin a dialogue. John Gray, in his book, *Men Are from Mars and Women Are from Venus*, talks about the need for communication between spouses. Conflict in any intimate relationship is inevitable. It is how a person deals with conflict that results in healthy or unhealthy consequences and the resultant toll it takes on the body. Effective stress management is essential to prevent coronary artery disease in both men and women.

In general, women have to take better care of themselves. If overweight, they need to lose weight. Simple, right? No, I know it is not simple, but I have so many examples of women who lose weight forever once they commit themselves to changes that lead them to a more accepting and healthy lifestyle.

Exercise and good eating habits are a must. Women need to be aware of their increased risk for heart disease after menopause and talk with their physician about estrogen replacement therapy. Women and men alike must stop smoking and practice effective stress management. Taking care of the heart is a lifelong strategy towards overall good health. Even before a child's birth, the health of the child is dependent on the mother's actions during pregnancy. Mom, the woman, the Goddess of Love and Sacrifice is the role model for the family. As a guardian of family's health she should encourage a healthy example of healthy shopping, healthy meals, and no smoking.

Prescription for Coronary Prevention and Reversal Program Rx

1. *Surya Namaskar*—every morning. Repeat five times.

2. *High Fiber Breakfast* including skim milk, oats and fruit.

3. *Power Lunch* including soup, yogurt, whole wheat bread, low fat cheese, cottage cheese and salad.

4. *High Protein Dinner* including beans, bread, pasta soya product. Fish, skinless breast of turkey or chicken and occasionally a lean piece of beef. All of them should be broiled or baked only.

5. *Aerobic Exercise* for 30 minutes a day at the prescribed aerobic level.

6. *Stress management* using relaxation techniques with emphasis on the realization of the idea that things usually work out, that most situations are not worth dying for.

7. *No Smoking. PERIOD.*

8. *Antioxidents with recommended dose of Vitamin. C and E and Folic acid daily.*

I will discuss this prescription in the next chapters. Before we go any further, I wish to repeat again that it is you alone who has control of your body. If you don't take control, nobody else will.

7

How to Manage Your Stress

"The rise of human loneliness may be one of the most serious sources of disease in the Twentieth Century."—James J. Lynch, Ph.D.

BEFORE I SAY ANYTHING ABOUT STRESS, LET me say that for 67 percent of the patients who came to our Cardiac Rehabilitation Center after a heart disease, the main cause of the disease is toxic stress (hostility, isolation, impulsiveness and a Type A personality). Stress is the most abused word in the English language. Let me share with you what I consider to be stress. Stress is the opposite of leisure, or the time one spends as one pleases. English author G. K. Chesterton defined leisure as being allowed to do nothing. Nowadays doing nothing is considered degrading and sinful.

In 1676 Hooke's law of physics, studied today by engineers, stated that the elastic limit is where the maximum stress can be sustained and still allow it to return to the original condition. Strain is proportional to stress. Selye, a physician, in 1950 defined *stress* as the nonspecific response of the body to change.

The stress I am talking about has nothing to do with physics or the "Law of Physics." Stress is discussed so casually that the word has lost its meaning and is being redefined almost every time the medical community has a chance to do so. Biochemists have joined the ranks now with a new term called "oxidative stress." Imagine how much stress is involved in defining the term "stress!"

Does *"Stress Test"* refer to the "stress" we are talking about? No, the *"stress test"* refers to the exercise procedure used to evaluate cardiovascular fitness. A "mental stress test" also may increase the heart rate, and this test may be more accurate in predicting a person who is prone to have a heart attack. To evaluate heart attack prone person, I use a computer program developed by Robert Eliot, MD, for evaluating mental stress, along with the physical stress test. This is done by checking the blood pressure and heart rate response to the short term adrenaline release stimulated by three different techniques and plotting the body's response to perceived threat.

Stress is perceived by and reacted to differently by individuals. As stress perception is different for each of us, the strategy to fight it is also variable. One person may react to stress by jogging and another by eating more or smoking or internalizing it. Most chronic problems in our body are thought to be stress related.

Half of the patients who come to my office have stress-related diseases. As I said before 67 percent of the patients in the Cardiac Rehabilitation Center have what I call toxic stress. A high percentage of our patients are in the rehabilitation program not because of major cholesterol problems but because of toxic stress, which results in behavior problems of overeating and other disorders.

We all know what stress is and how it feels to be "stressed out." It is safe to say that anyone who is alive has most likely felt stress at one time or another. For many people, stress is an ongoing daily occurrence. Since almost everyone experiences stress, it is important to know how to handle stress and how to gain control over our stress inducing activities.

Being Type A is not enough to make you prone to coronary artery disease. I know of so many Type A people who are CEOs of different companies who do not have heart disease. How we *perceive* the stress is more important than that we have it. A study by Ortho Gomer showed that 17.3 percent of **socially integrated** Type A CEOs had coronary artery disease compared to 20.9 percent of **socially integrated** Type B CEOs. But for those CEOs who where **socially isolated** the results were quite different: 68.9 percent of **socially isolated** Type A CEOs had heart disease compare to 43.8 percent of **socially isolated** Type B CEOs.

This shows that people who are isolated, either Type A or Type B, have increased risk of coronary artery disease. If you have a Type A personality and you stay isolated and don't share your emotions with anybody, keeping problems to yourself, then you are in trouble. Isolation with anger and hostility makes you a **"Type H."** I hope to share with you how you can determine if you have a "Type H" personality and what steps you need to take to help yourself.

As a kid when I would get angry my grandma would always say, "Go drink a glass of water first, and then say what you want to say." At that time her advice did not make much sense to me, but it does now. By weight our brains are 75 percent water. When you are mad or stressed out, your brain uses up more water, which you need to replace to let your brain cells process the mega information without messing up the outcome (like getting confused). On average you lose ten cups of water a day, and if you are sweating you lose even more and you need to drink more. Just before giving your first commencement speech you are so nervous that you have to drink water just before walking to the podium, or you will take a glass of water to the podium. Whenever you are under stress your brain needs more water so that the cells can transfer the messages clearly and objectively. It is important to remember that by getting mad and stressed out you are only hurting yourself physically and mentally. Grandma was right on this as she was with her advice to eat more greens and broccoli.

Before I became aware of my heart problems, I was often intolerant. If I became angry, I bottled up my anger because I believed that it was useless to try to change my personality. I wanted to hide my anger from the outside world. When I would get angry at certain situations in the hospital, I kept it inside. If you asked most of the nurses at the hospital, they would say that I never got angry. My family, however, would tell you a different story.

Hostility and anger will harm your heart. A sudden onset of anger doubles the risk of a heart attack in the next two hours. Hostility and anger are two aspects of Type A behavior that we call **Type H behavior**, which is considered to be pathological.

If you are a hot reactor, as Dr. Eliot refers to those people who show extreme bodily reactions to stress, you are releasing powerful chemicals such as adrenaline and cortisol into your bloodstream. Over time these substances damage your heart. Not all hot reactors are Type A personalities. However, people who habitually overreact to stress incur wide fluctuations in their blood pressures. If you feel that you are often in the "fight or flight" mode, you could be a hot reactor.

My father used to tell me that being a physician was a noble profession. He told me that I needed to give 100 percent to my patients. He believed that sitting down and talking and listening to patients would take away half of their ailments. My patients came to see me so that I could solve their problems, not so they could solve mine.

I remember that a couple of times I even canceled my vacation because one of my patients was extremely ill. I thought that if I would leave town something might happen to my patient. If I did go anywhere, I would call my office and check on my patients to see how they were doing. Basically I did not trust anyone, and I was never relaxed. I was fearful, and I kept the fear and anger hidden away inside of me and would take it out on my family when I got home. Instead of simply hiding my anger, which I thought I was doing at work, I was unleashing it inside me. Anger was eating away at me, specifically at my heart.

When you have been angry or on an emotional, mental, or physical overload all day, you take it home with you in the form of stress. At night when you are stressed and your mind is working overtime as a result of all the stress that you have internalized throughout the day, your body cannot relax, and you cannot sleep. In the morning when you get up, your body releases cortisol and increases it throughout the day until evening when the level in your body starts to drop allowing your body to relax and sleep. However, if you do not sleep, your body releases more cortisol to keep up your functional capacity. The constant release of cortisol eventually can be detrimental to your health because of its toxic nature. Over time, cortisol may cause injury to the interior lining of your arteries, known as the endothelium. Platelets collect at the site of the injured arterial wall, and cholesterol will start to build up until it slowly closes the artery. In chronic stress your body will continue to make cortisol even though it is harmful, and your heart will end up paying the price for the daily, weekly, monthly, and yearly accumulation of stress.

How do you control your emotions and manage your stress? One thing you should remember is that whatever event occurs to cause you stress is not the problem. Rather, it is how you *react* to that event or stress.

Although I was advised to meditate as one of the way to relieve and manage stress, I could not take this route. I just could not sit still and concentrate long enough to meditate. I could not stay focused. I would close my eyes, but within a few minutes my mind would take off and visit all those places where I would prefer not to go, actually causing more stress and strain. Fortunately for me, just at that time I got exposed to a wonderful teacher, Robert Eliot, MD, who experienced heart disease himself when he was only 40 years old. He recognized stress as being his main problem and decided to devote his life to learning and teaching the relationship between stress and heart disease. He was instrumental in helping me to identify and modify my personal behavior by relaxation technique and self-talk. I found this to be more helpful than sitting for an hour to meditate which I could not do it anyway.

Robert Eliot in his books, *Is It Worth Dying For?* and *From Stress to Strength*, talks about the *ABC*s of stress management. According to Eliot, *A* is the ***Accentuating*** event, *B* is your ***Belief*** system—which is the major driver of stress management—and finally, *C* is the ***Consequence***.

As he said it is not the event which is the problem but how you react to the event with your belief system. Let me relate to you an incident from my life and share with you how I reacted at that time and how I would respond to that same situation now. I am sure some of you may be in the same shoes as I was.

A, the Accentuating Event. My wife, kids and I were returning from Dayton to Urbana, a small beautiful town where I used to practice medicine, to see one of my patients who was in the hospital. My wife asked me if we could stop at a department store on the way home. She told me that it would take her only five minutes to make her purchase. Reluctantly I agreed and told her that I was going to hold her to her promise. As I sat in the car waiting for her, five minutes lapsed into thirty-five minutes. This was **A**, the Accentuating event. (Many of you who are reading this probably already are thinking that a spouse's proposed five-minute trip into a department store is unrealistic, if not comical, in the first place.)

B, the Belief. I believed that she would return within five minutes. When she did not appear within the five minute time frame, I began my self-talk. I started with negative self-talk. My self-pitying monologue encompassed thoughts that she did not care about me or my patients. It really started bothering me that she had seemingly broke her promise and I felt that I could not trust her. As my negative self-talk continued, and my wife had still not returned to the car, I became angrier and angrier.

C, the Consequence. When my wife returned to the car thirty minutes late, I was so angry that I began yelling at her as soon as she opened the car door. Her response was to begin yelling at me. My yelling at her had prompted her reaction. As a result of the misunderstanding, we did not speak to each other for two or three days. Finally, when we did start speaking, she told me what had happened in the store. She related that when she went to pay for her purchase, the computer did not work properly, and the sales people had to fix it. The repair took about fifteen minutes and caused her unexplained delay. She could not leave that place because her check was stuck in his printer.

As it turned out, my belief system was not wrong, but how I reacted to it was. I should have been having positive self-talk instead of a negative one. I should have told myself that something unexpected must have arisen. Instead of flying off the handle, I should have given her time to explain what had happened. If I had used positive self-talk, I might have been somewhat annoyed at her delay, but not to the point that I would have exploded upon seeing her. I would have realized that she really does care about me, my feelings, and my patients. And had I not exploded, the consequence of our not speaking to each other for a couple of days would most likely have turned out quite differently.

After discussing this with Dr. Eliot, I realized that handling stress in a positive manner was the most important thing that I needed to do. I began working with this simple technique of self talk rather than trying to do meditation when I was angry. Meditation and exercise also have their roles to play, but in these situations the self talk is the best way to handle the event. I learned the *ABC* technique of managing stress and used it on every occasion when I found myself getting angry. Working on my positive belief system and incorporating positive self-talk have helped me change the way I approach stressful situations and have allowed me to manage stress successfully. It is important for everyone to emphasize the positive side of self-talk especially under stress-producing situations.

Using the *ABC* approach with my teenage children has improved our relationship. It is helpful to know that we can be in control of our feelings and our actions. It is usually our actions that cause others to react to us in a positive or negative manner. Many times people are only following our lead. If we get angry inappropriately and act in a hostile way towards others, are we not in fact giving others the green light to react to us in a similar manner?

I have developed another important guideline in my life. During anger the normal body reaction to the fight or flight response is that it will release adrenaline and pump the heart to provide up to 300 percent more blood to the peripheral muscle cells to fight the danger that the body system had sensed. This starts an alarm system which may be harmful to the body. In such a situation I usually ask myself if this situation is worth dying for. I get upset only if I really think that it is worth it. Otherwise I just drink a glass of water, count up to ten and try to rationalize the event using my **A B** and **C**s. Self talk is worth working on. I can assure you that this procedure will help you gain control of your life events. I did it; you can do it too.

Before starting this program I was resistant to changes. I was stressed easily and had a Type A personality. I was very impulsive and had quite a bit of hostility associated with depression. When you are angry and under stress all the time, you use up all your adrenaline. Afterwards a natural body reaction is to be depressed so that the body can charge itself for the next episode of anger. This swinging nature of your body causes most of the harm because of the exposure to toxic stress.

Additional ways to manage stress include doing those things that make you feel relaxed. Some people might practice yoga or another type of meditation or exercise. For others, taking a walk, talking to a friend, or listening to music might help them unwind. Or simply sitting down to read a book or watch television might help. Most people know what makes them feel better and feel less tense.

Whatever works for you to reduce and relieve your stress is your key to stress management. Practicing stress management will help you gain control over your emotions and relieve your tension. By changing your beliefs and engaging in positive self-talk, you can learn to react in a positive manner, instead of a negative one. Stress will not magically disappear from your life, but you can learn how to deal with it in non self-destructive ways. And, as a result of having developed better self-control over your emotions, you will improve your relationships with others.

Ultimately it is you and only you who is responsible for your own health.

Nobody else will do it for you. If you know that toxic stress is the cause of your disease, then it is incumbent upon you to take care of yourself using these techniques. I recommend that you read the books written by Robert Eliot "Is it worth dying for?" I also recommend that you use a relaxation technique for about fifteen to twenty minutes a day.

The Mental Imagery Meditation and Relaxation Process

I have used this technique to help me manage day-to-day stress.

I started using the process when I could not do meditation sitting in one place for more than a few minutes. I have found it to be useful and practical, since I can use it any place, anytime. Once you start employing this technique regularly you, too, can use it at anytime.

To start with you need to sit down in a comfortable position. You may even want to lie down on a comfortable mattress. Make sure that you are warm enough and that your clothes are comfortable.

1. Close your eyes, relax and breathe normally to allow the process of performing direct visualization to massage the physical and mental stress out of your body.

2. Let your jaw muscle relax, allowing your jaw to slowly drop creating a little opening between the upper and the lower jaw.

3. Let your shoulders muscles relax and then let your shoulder hang down as if they have no support.

4. Become aware of your breathing. Breathe in a long deep breath through your nose and let it out through your mouth. Do this a couple of times.

5. Now concentrate on the pineal gland, which is between your eyes and about two inches deep inside your brain, and try to relax.

6. Keep breathing like this for about three to five minutes or till you feel comfortable. Pay attention to the warmth of your air as you are breathing in and breathing out.

7. Progressively and systematically beginning with your feet, relax your leg, arm, upper body and neck until your body is limp like a rag doll.

8. Keep like this as long as you feel comfortable. Concentrate on your breathing and keep your jaw relaxed.

9. When you feel that you are ready to get up, open your eyes slowly and start breathing normally.

10. Slowly get up and be ready to go back to whatever you were doing. All the tension will be gone, you will be more connected and you will be all charged up to do more and with better vigor now as you are full of energy and happiness.

I use this technique whenever I have a conflict going on in myself, whenever I am stressed out or whenever I am unable to sleep. You can use this technique as many times a day as you want. In certain situations I also have modified this to a one-minute routine to calm me down such as a few minutes before giving a lecture to a new group.

8

Smoking and Alcohol

**"When you have a choice and don't make it,
that is in itself a choice."—William James.**

SMOKING IS A HARMFUL, ADDICTIVE HABIT THAT
contributes to 300,000 deaths a year in the United States.
Smokers are about ten times more likely to develop lung
cancer than nonsmokers and twice as likely to develop heart
disease. Smoking a pack a day will shorten a person's life by
about six years. On average, a thirty-five year old male lives
about 2.3 years longer if he quits smoking, and a female
will live about 2.8 years longer. Cigarette smoking is the
leading cause of cardiovascular deaths.

Twenty minutes after your last cigarette, blood pressure
and pulse rates drop. After eight hours without smoking,
carbon monoxide levels in your blood return to normal, and
the body's oxygen level is restored. After twenty-four hours,
the chance of having a heart attack decreases. Two days after the last cigarette, the nerve endings in your nose resume
growth, enhancing your senses of smell and taste. Seventy-
two hours later, the bronchial tubes in your lungs start to
relax, and you can breathe much easier. Within two weeks

to three months, your circulation improves, and you can walk easily without becoming short of breath. Your lung function is much better, and, within one to nine months, your overall energy level increases, and your lungs become clearer.

After five years without smoking, your chance of dying from lung cancer decreases from 137 to 72 per 100,000 people. After ten years, it decreases to 12 per 100,000 people, the rate for nonsmokers. Other cancers also decrease.

So why doesn't everyone just quit smoking? Quitting is very difficult, but not impossible. Cigarettes and other forms of tobacco contain the addictive drug, nicotine. The pharmacological and behavioral processes that determine addiction to tobacco are similar to those of other addictive drugs. Nicotine has definite mind and mood altering effects. It is a stimulant that improves the user's attention span and concentration. Overcoming an established dependence on nicotine is more difficult than overcoming alcohol or heroin dependence.

Behavior modification is the key to breaking the addiction. A person needs to be trained and empowered to stop smoking. Medications also can help cut back on smoking until the addiction is broken.

Smoking speeds up metabolism. Smokers usually burn 100 to 200 calories a day from smoking. People who quit smoking often develop a sweet tooth. Because people who quit smoking usually gain weight, they fear gaining weight, especially women.

Women, on average, smoke fewer cigarettes than men, but women usually have a harder time quitting. No one is sure about the difference in social and psychological pressures between men and women to quit smoking, but fear of getting fat is certainly a factor among women in their reluctance to stop smoking. Many women who have stopped smoking start smoking again once they begin to gain weight even though they know that the consequences of smoking are far more serious than for weight gain.

If you want to stop smoking, join a support group. You need to prepare yourself psychologically in advance to avoid smoking when the temptation arises. It is important to keep busy and use a substitute such as sugar-free gum, mints, or carrot and celery strips if you feel the need to have something in your mouth. Avoid places where people smoke. Go to restaurants that prohibit smoking and to public places such as museums and libraries. Avoid people who smoke and tell friends and relatives that you no longer allow smoking in your home. Stay away from co-workers who smoke on coffee breaks. If you have more than two drinks a day, reduce the amount of alcohol you drink, because many people associate smoking with drinking. Keep mints in your pocket for when you feel the need to smoke. And try relaxation techniques to help you unwind instead of reaching for a cigarette.

Why go to all the trouble to quit smoking? You will feel better, regain your sense of taste and smell, lose the odor of stale tobacco that lingers on your breath, clothes, and hair, have fewer respiratory problems and illnesses, and be more energetic. You are more likely to live longer and be in better health throughout your life. And you will help provide those you love with the opportunity to breathe smoke-free air.

Alcohol: Does it really Prevent Heart Disease?

Whenever I am presenting a lecture about prevention of heart disease, someone will ask, "Can a drink a day keep the heart attack away?" The answer appears to be yes, but only when alcohol is drunk in moderate amounts.

An old Russian saying is: "Drink a glass of wine after your soup and you steal the ruble from the doctor." Everybody in Europe and Russia knew about this, but the secret was leaked out to the American public by CBS's 60 minutes news segment on "French Paradox" a few years ago. Americans seized the message and promptly headed for the liquor stores and the fruit market to buy wine—and apples, since we knew the saying, "An apple a day keeps the doctor away." Now we were introduced to another saying that wine will steal the ruble, all of this in the name of health. Wine stocks went up and so did the consumption of alcohol.

At the same time the world's medical researchers went to work and came back with numerous studies on the diverse populations showing that "moderate alcohol consumption is associated with a significantly decreased incidents of death due to coronary heart disease." The main message was that moderate alcohol consumption, which means one or two glasses of alcohol a day, will decrease heart disease. The studies also confirmed that when it comes to alcohol, more is not better and actually may be detrimental for the heart.

We in the physician community were very uncomfortable with the idea that there is something good to say about alcohol. Most of us are afraid that educating patients about potential benefits of moderate drinking will encourage them to drink more and promote alcoholism. Actually, heavy alcohol users have a number of cardiovascular problems including enlarged heart, high blood pressure, and irregular heart beat. We also know that heavy alcohol users are often also smokers and that combination increases the chance of lung cancer and breast cancer.

Although conservative about alcohol prescribed as medicine, I answer this favorite question ("Can a drink a day keep the heart attack away?") saying that I strongly believe that it is not the wine consumption only but the social interaction associated with it that explains why the incidence of death from heart disease is low in a wine consuming society. The Monica heart study, which was a study of heart disease in twenty-one European countries, found that the incidence of heart disease was low in countries where people consumed alcohol as well as a lot of fresh fruits and vegetables.

Is it simply the wine in the French diet that gives them protection against cardiovascular disease? Or is it a combination of wine and lifestyle? The French eat a leisurely main meal, including wine, with friends in the middle of the day in a relaxed atmosphere. The French usually dine at regular intervals at a leisurely pace in a tranquil ambiance and usually with social interaction among friends and family. Wine in Europe is consumed as food. They sip, swish, and swallow the wine. They usually eat their larger meal at lunch and do not snack between. How about us Americans? We usually eat fast food on the run and often alone. The average time between ordering, serving, consuming, and leaving the fast food restaurant is about 210 seconds. Just imagine how therapeutic wine and food could be in this fast-paced life.

The next popular question that people usually ask is if red wine is superior to white wine. The answer is, I think so. Alcohol in any form has an euphoric effect, relaxes you, and slows down your adrenaline release. But the real explanation seems to be in complex chemical substances such as fungicides, flavanoids, polyphenols and resveratrol. All of these are fancy long names are known in simpler language as antioxidants which prevent LDL or oxidized cholesterol from damaging the inside of the artery, causing plaque formation and obstruction.

Resveratrol (fungus on the skin of the grapes) and catechin are powerful antioxidants that combat coronary artery disease. People are trying to focus on these compounds to see if they can make and sell them as a nutritional supplements. "Life in the fast lane!" "A pill to cure anything." I can't imagine why one would rather take a pill than drink red wine.

Red wine is actually a preserved whole fruit that contains skin, juice, and seeds. The combination provides us with such natural antioxidants as phenolics, catechin and resveratrol. White wine also delivers antioxidants, but not that many. Phenolics are natural antioxidants that protect the body from the process of oxidation, which causes all kinds of chronic diseases. The phenolics are more effective in slowing down the LDL oxidation than even vitamin C or E. Did you know that onions have the same number of phenolics as the grape skin? Just some "food for thought" for wine drinkers.

While any alcohol reduces the clumping together of platelets, red wine appears to have superior properties in that regard due to its flavanoids, polyphenols, and a fungicide on the skin of the red grape which inhibits the oxidation of LDL cholesterol. White wine does not produce the same effect because the skin of the grape is removed prior to crushing. However, one study, comparing California Chardonnay (white grape) to Cabernet Sauvignon (red grape), found that the Chardonnay was superior in its effects on lipids and antioxidants. Would grape juice have the same beneficial properties? It appears that it might have some beneficial effect, but not to the same degree as wine.

Before I go ahead and give you the prescription for drinking wine, I must share with you a word of caution. People who drink too much alcohol have a greater chance of mouth, throat, and esophageal cancer and liver diseases. Women metabolize alcohol slower than men. That's why women are recommended not to have more than one drink a day. To receive cardiovascular benefits from alcohol, moderation is the key—one drink a day. It is important for women of childbearing age to remember that even moderate alcohol consumption can have adverse effects on a fetus and can lead to fetal alcohol syndrome. Also drinking more than one drink a day has been linked to an increased risk of breast cancer.

Just a note about hard liquor, beer, and wine. People who consume beer and hard liquor have three times the risk of developing a large stomach, a "beer belly," compared to wine drinkers. Beer belly people have larger waists than hips, and it is a medically proven fact that if your waist and hip ratio is more than 0.8, your chance of heart disease is greater.

Finally, let me share with you a little more about the research done in this field of alcohol and the mechanism by which it may be helping us. A University of Pittsburgh study on 128 people tracking the effects of moderate drinking found an increase of ten to twenty percent in estradiol, an estrogenic hormone. Estrogen is associated with an increase in high density lipoproteins or HDL, the good cholesterol, which is responsible for removing LDL cholesterol from the endothelium, the lining of arterial walls.

The Boston Physician Health Study demonstrated that moderate alcohol intake increased the level of the tissue plasminogen activator, TPA. This naturally produced chemical in the blood prevents blood from clotting. Doctors who drank one or two drinks a day had a 30 percent to 40 percent lower incidence of heart disease.

A British study following about 12,000 middle-aged physicians for thirteen years found a similarly protective effect on the heart with moderate alcohol intake among those who had one or two drinks a day. However, they found that if a larger quantity of alcohol was regularly consumed, the mortality rate increased. Any protective effect from alcohol is lost by consuming large quantities.

How does alcohol affect the heart? Ethyl alcohol in any form will increase the HDL cholesterol, and the higher the HDL cholesterol, the lower the risk of coronary artery disease. Various studies have suggested that about fifty percent of alcohol's cardioprotective effect is attained through its effect on HDL cholesterol. Moderate and heavy alcohol consumption raises HDL cholesterol levels. The subfractions of HDL, HDL2 and HDL3 are affected by alcohol consumption, and evidence suggests that both subfractions have a protective effect on the heart. Alcohol also increases the level of Lipoprotein A1 and A2. They are associated with the formation of the HDL particle, and alcohol has an antithrombotic effect that may be cardioprotective. The antithrombotic property of alcohol increases the thromboxane ratio and decreases the thickness of platelets which reduces clotting. Alcohol actually increases the endogenous tissue type of plasminogen activator.

It cannot be oversimplified that the maximum amount of alcohol is *one* drink a day for cardiovascular purposes. For some people in American society, the idea of drinking alcohol is a complex issue. Alcohol can be an addictive drug and is widely abused, ranking second only to tobacco usage. The abuse of alcohol is responsible for about 10,000 deaths a year, and the problem of drunken driving concerns everyone. For these reasons, although a moderate amount of alcohol may be healthy for the heart, prophylactic use of alcohol has remains controversial. Moderate alcohol usage appears to be safe and beneficial for the heart in people who are not alcoholics or have other problems related to alcohol consumption.

My final answer to the question "to drink or not to drink?" is simple: **you be the judge.**

9

Aerobic Exercise

I know that if I could prescribe exercise in the form of a PILL I would be an instant millionaire.—N. Saini.

SOMETIME BETWEEN CHILDHOOD AND ADUlthood, the fun seems to go out of exercise for many people. Children regard exercise as play while most adults think of it as work. Mention the word exercise to an adult and the negative responses vary from "I don't like to exercise" to "I don't have time" to "It's boring."

A wealth of data available from different studies for the last many years has a simple message :

Don't be a couch potato. Turn off the television and spend half an hour to an hour every day walking, jogging, playing tennis, riding a bicycle, or mowing the lawn. The famous saying, "Use it or lose it," fits the exercise philosophy perfectly.

It does not matter if you are 40 or 70; not exercising on a regular basis is detrimental to your health. Exercise, no matter how you view it, is beneficial to your health. Ancient Greek, Roman and Indian literature will testify to that.

I remember a conversation which took place during my discussion with one of my patients who asked me why he should exercise. Curious about his question I answered back with another question, "Why not?"

With a big smile on his face he presented to me a recent article published in a newspaper quoting a recent study done on exercise on Harvard University alumni. The summary report of the article showed that the exercising group lived on average only two years longer then the general population. They exercised on average 30 minutes a day, and if you totaled all the hours that they exercised throughout this study, the total came to about two and a half years. According to his analysis, he would waste valuable time spent exercising because the net gain would be nothing. Spending two and a half years of cumulative exercise time to gain only two years in his lifetime did not make any sense to him. He did not want to kill himself with the stress and torture of exercising and said he would rather live two fewer years.

He had a rather strong argument for which I was not well prepared. After getting my thoughts together and becoming angry at press reports that are released to the media causing confusion and harm to the general public, I started explaining to him and his wife why he should exercise. His wife had no problem understanding my reasons, but he was trying to pull every trick to get out of exercising.

I explained to him that a person is not exercising to prolong one's life, but to improve the *quality of life* and that is all. The last year of our lives we spend about 60 percent of the total medical care dollars that we will spend through out our lifetime. If we exercise regularly we will prevent not only heart disease and its complications, but all the other chronic diseases such as osteoarthritis, high blood pressure, diabetes and obesity. Not only will we feel better, we also are helping to have a good quality of life.

There are many mornings when we do not want to get out of the bed to exercise. Then we push ourselves because we know that we are going to be rewarded afterwards by feeling good, and it surely happens that way. After exercising because of the release of endorphins and other happy hormones in our bodies, we feel like million-dollar persons.

The trick is to exercise only in the *aerobic level*. (I will explain later on what I mean by "aerobic level.") So I told my patient that he needs to exercise not only to prevent the recurrence of heart disease but also to enjoy the good quality of life and prevent those mammoth medical bills. He smiled, looked at his wife and said, "Honey, I don't think I can get out of this."

This conversation took place in 1992 and ever since this person has been exercising regularly in our center. He is one of our mentors now, a person I call upon when I need to convince a patient why he or she should exercise or to explain the extent of the payback once a person gets hooked into taking care of his or her body by exercising and making other lifestyle changes. If you are in the same predicament as Joe was, no more posturing! Get out of that chair and start exercising for a good quality of life.

Quality of life! What does it mean? Quality of life means that you are enjoying living in the present moment. You can enjoy yourself only if you are physically and mentally connected. You have quality of life if you are able to smile, work, converse with pleasure and effectiveness, if you are mentally clear, able to take care of yourself and not dependent on anybody for the care of your body.

I am not afraid of death; I had a very close call and am completely convinced that the good Lord is the only one who knows when my time is coming. Once I was able to convince myself of this fact and was able to accept it as a fact, then I decided to do everything I could in my power to have a good quality of life. I want to go home smiling, without prolonging my life with these wonders of modern medicine and fancy medical gadgets or crippled by stroke or an incapacitating heart attack. I am not against nursing homes. For those who need to be in them they are fine, but I will do everything I can to keep myself out of them. A nursing home stay would wipe out my savings and, in the process, any small inheritance my kids may be entitled to receive.

Once you have heart disease you have a good chance of getting it again. Exercise is an integral part of the lifestyle changes you must adopt to prevent the recurrences. As I said before I am not afraid of death, but I am scared of getting a stroke. My intention is not to compete with the Lord, but to complement Him and do what I am supposed to do. I found out that the answer was simple. It was exercising religiously at the proper aerobic level, along with managing my stress and eating heart healthy food. You have to have a strong conviction and mission to exercise and make the proper lifestyle changes to avoid this deadly disease.

Exercise, as I said, no matter how you view it, is beneficial. It is important to know how the body functions in order to understand how exercise helps the body. Imagine that your body is a car. A car cannot run without fuel. Just as there are different grades of gasoline (unleaded, unleaded plus, premium) that an engine can burn to make the car run, the body runs on different types of fuel depending on the length and the degree of energy needed for any given activity.

The food that we eat is turned into fuel for the body. Gasoline is measured by the gallon. The foods we consume are measured by calories. Foods with a high fat content have the most calories per gram; a gram of fat contains nine calories. The food that we eat is turned into glucose, or sugar, and it is contained within each cell of the body. Our bodies need a certain number of calories every day to stay alive. The number of calories that the body needs to maintain itself depends upon the age, weight, height, and sex of the person. Men need more calories than women to maintain body function. (See page 120 for a formula to calculate your Basal Metabolism Rate, which helps you determine how many calories you need to maintain your weight.)

In addition to body maintenance, a person needs to consume enough food each day equal to the energy required for the level of activities performed. If a person's intake of food, as measured in calories, is equal to the energy expended in a day, the person will remain at the same weight. If a person's intake of food is less than the energy used, a person will lose weight. However, if a person takes in more calories than are needed for one's daily activities, the person will experience a gain in weight as those calories, not needed by the body, are stored as fat.

To perform any body movement like walking, running, or sitting our body needs energy. Our body is a beautiful computer. It controls the amount and form of energy released at different activity levels. If you are walking slowly the body uses one form of energy. If you are running it uses a different form of energy. This energy is released by a complex biochemical reaction that our body computer helps perform to provide the right type of fuel. The most efficient form of energy is released when you body is performing at the *aerobic level.*

Let me explain what I mean by "aerobic level." I am sure you have heard the term "aerobics" by now. Aerobics is an advertising term used to encourage you to exercise. Technically, however, "aerobic" refers to the level at which your body utilizes glucose, fat and oxygen to provide you with energy. At the aerobic level, your body is obtaining 70 percent of its energy from fat and 30 percent from sugar. At aerobic level the body is releasing the good hormone known as endorphin and a natural clot buster known as "tpa." Endorphin is chemically similar to morphine, which is why you always feel better after aerobic exercise. Your body's natural internal medicine is working here.

Endorphin also seems to control the cementing capability of clot-happy blood platelets. This is important because sixty to eighty percent of heart attacks are caused by a fresh clot in the artery that clogs the blood supply to that part of the heart's muscle. This blood clot happens because the platelet adheres to the fissure caused by a rupture of the plaque, resulting in clotting up the artery.

That is why we ask patients to take an aspirin as soon as they think they are having a heart attack. The aspirin thins the blood so that it will not clot. Of course, if you are exercising regularly, the endorphin your body releases will keep the platelets under check.

The aerobic level is different for every person. We calculate this by doing a special VO_2 Stress test. For this test the patient is exercised on the treadmill while breathing only through a tube in his or her mouth. A computer calculates the exact aerobic level of that person by checking the exchange of oxygen and carbon dioxide. After calculating this, we prescribe an aerobic range for that person so that he or she can get the maximum benefit out of the exercise.

A simpler way of calculating the target aerobic heart rate is detailed in page 117. When you are exercising at the aerobic level, your body will utilize energy from the complex biochemical reaction using fat, glucose and oxygen as the main ingredients. If you are exercising below the aerobic level, as in taking a leisurely stroll, the body will utilize energy from the biochemical reaction of glucose and oxygen. If you are exercising at an anaerobic level, that is using the energy from the biochemical reaction using sugar and protein without using oxygen, the body will release energy which you can't use for a long period of time.

Our beautiful body provides energy for different types of activity that we are performing. If you keep exercising at the anaerobic level (as we used to say, "no pain no gain") then you will burn most of your energy from muscle and only a part from fat. As a matter of fact only 30 percent of fat is being burnt while 70 percent of sugar is being burnt at this level. As a result you lose more muscle than fat. And when you gain the weight back you gain fat more than muscle. This type of yo-yo weight gain is not only unhealthy, but also dangerous. You need muscle to burn fat. If you are burning muscle, then what will burn the fat?

Prolonged exercise that elevates the heart rate and causes a person to breathe deeply over a sustained period of time is known as aerobic ("with oxygen") exercise. Aerobic exercise burns more calories than anaerobic exercise and helps a person develop stamina. In addition, the more intense or vigorous the "aerobic activity" is, the more calories the body burns in response to the level of physical activity. This is why a person burns more calories playing handball than walking.

To lose weight through exercise, a person must reach the aerobic level for a continuous period of at least fifteen minutes twice a day. Since the body is accustomed to burning glucose, or sugar, as the fuel to provide energy to the body, it is reluctant to burn the fat stored in fat cells for energy. Regular aerobic exercise is the best way to burn fat.

As previously discussed, a buildup of fatty deposits in the coronary arteries is what causes atherosclerosis, or hardening of the arteries. This fatty buildup restricts blood flow to the heart and results in coronary artery disease which increases a person's risk for heart attack. Aerobic exercise is a good preventive measure to reduce the buildup of fatty deposits, or lipids, in the coronary arteries.

When a person begins to exercise regularly at the aerobic level, the body recognizes that the person is exercising and starts to burn fat as well as glucose. The energy delivered to the body from burning glucose and fat makes adenosine triphosphate (ATP). The adenosine triphosphate contracts the muscles. It is through the contraction of the muscles that the body burns fat.

And thus the cycle is repeated.

If a person is not exercising at the aerobic level, the body will not make ATP, which contracts the muscles allowing the body to burn fat. When glucose in muscle tissue burns, it is broken down into a chemical known as pyruvate. If there is enough oxygen in the muscle, the pyruvate is converted into carbon dioxide and water and is released through the lungs upon exhalation. If there is not enough oxygen, the glucose is not completely metabolized, producing less energy than if it were completely metabolized. The pyruvate turns into lactic acid in the muscle, and the excess lactic acid is deposited in the bloodstream. The lactic acid impairs muscle contraction and will eventually stop muscles from contracting. Symptoms of lactic acid buildup in the muscles include muscle cramping and shortness of breath. Lactic acid is a by-product of anaerobic exercise—exercise "without oxygen." However, the body can change lactic acid back into glucose as the person takes in more oxygen and activity is performed at the aerobic level.

Therefore, to lose weight, a person must consistently exercise at the aerobic level for a minimum of fifteen minutes twice a day to direct the body to burn fat in addition to glucose. Once the aerobic activity has been established on a regular basis, the body builds up muscle with this mode of activity and these muscles become an efficient fat-burning machines. Remember our body has trillions of cells, and each cell can become efficient in burning fat.

It is extremely important for people trying to lose weight to give their bodies enough time to recognize aerobic exercise. The body needs to learn to burn fat. As the person progressively exercises at the aerobic level and develops a routine, the body burns more fat. The keys to aerobic exercise are consistency and continuity. Consistency—three to five times a week; and continuity—sustained aerobic exercise for a minimum of fifteen minutes.

You cannot just exercise for two weeks and then expect to lose the pounds you have managed to gain over the past several years, and you are certainly not going to lose weight if your exercise program is not consistent. Your body is very smart. Once your body realizes you are person who will exercise a few days and then stop, it thinks, "Why should I waste my energy teaching my cells to become efficient fat-burning machines? After a while this person is going to stop exercising anyway." Not only are you giving in to laziness, but you have also trained your cells in the same way.

So if you are really interested in losing weight, remember these two Cs: **Consistency and Continuity.** You will need to keep exercising for at least four to six weeks before your cells begin to get the message that you are serious. They will then pass the word on to all their "buddy" cells to becomes efficient fat-burning cells. Once they get the message you are on your way to losing weight and feeling better.

Aerobic exercise, cycling, walking at a pace that increases the heart rate, jogging, swimming, etc., all increase a person's lung capacity, resulting in the ability to take in more oxygen. This produces more energy and strengthens the heart muscle, allowing it to perform more efficiently. It also burns up excess fat, the enemy that contributes to heart disease and cancer. Other benefits of aerobic exercise include an increase in the body's level of HDL, which carries harmful cholesterol out of the blood stream, a reduction in LDL (low density lipoprotein, the bad cholesterol), and a reduction in blood pressure, a risk factor in heart disease, kidney failure, and stroke.

Aerobic exercise can also help women prevent osteoporosis as weight bearing bones become stronger through physical activity. Physiologically, aerobic exercise increases the production of endorphins, the body's natural chemicals to reduce stress and stabilize moods. In addition, exercise enhances a sense of well-being by reducing tension and improving endurance. Overall, aerobic exercise plays a key role in maximizing a person's energy level and keeping the body, especially the heart and lungs, in good physical condition and the mind alert.

One of the best aerobic exercises is walking. It is a safe, simple, inexpensive, and beneficial exercise that a person can do alone or with others. Walking burns as many calories per mile as running. Studies have shown that a regimen of walking about nine miles per week can significantly prolong life. Walking boosts the immune response and improves circulation.

For walking to be effective, you must walk fast enough to increase your heart rate and walk for at least thirty minutes. When walking, keep your head and back straight and stomach muscles tight. Let your arms swing freely at your side. Take a long, comfortable stride and breathe deeply. If you have been inactive for a long time, you need to start slowly and gradually increase speed and distance. You can begin by walking fifteen minutes in the morning and fifteen minutes in the evening working up to forty-five minutes to one hour in either the morning or evening.

A good way to determine the pace of walking in the aerobic level is to talk with someone while walking. If you are out of breath or cannot maintain a conversation, you are walking too fast. Walk at your own pace and do not feel as if you have to compete with others by trying to walk at their pace.

Remember to warm up before walking by doing some simple stretches such as calf stretches, thigh stretches, and hamstring stretches, and a body stretch. See the diagram on page 118 for a recommended exercise warmup routine. It is also important to cool down after a walk that increases your heart rate by slowing the pace near the end of the walk and stretching as in the warm up.

The only equipment needed for walking is a good pair of walking shoes to provide comfort and support. The heel should be one half to three quarters of an inch higher than the sole and have arch support.

A good time to walk is before dinner as exercise curbs hunger. Another good time to walk is early in the morning before work. In bad weather, many people choose to walk in malls or in neighborhood schools if that option exists.

As stated previously, exercise will strengthen the heart, increase lung capacity, and provide more energy. Everyone should exercise within the target heart rate as determined by age. A person who is not used to exercising should start at the lower end of the target heart rate.

The recommended training heart rate is 60 percent to 80 percent of the maximum number of beats that your heart can beat in a minute. To figure your target heart rate, use the following formula:

Formula for Determining Target Heart Rate

Start with 220
— (subtract) your age
x 0.6 = lower end of target heart range
x 0.8 = higher end of target heart rate

Example
220
— 60 (age) = 160

160 x 0.6 = 96 beats per minute, the lower end of the target heart rate for a healthy 60-year-old person

160 x 0.8 = 128 beats per minute, the higher end of the target heart rate for a healthy 60-year-old person

---

Exercise does *not* have to hurt to be beneficial. Exercise is also habit forming. Once you have established a routine of walking, you will look forward to the exercise and feel better as a result of it.

The following table can help you calculate minutes per mile and miles per hour for walking.

Walking Speed Conversion Table

Steps per minute	Minutes per mile	Miles per hour
70	30	2.0
90	24	2.5
106	20	3.0
120	17	3.5
140	16	4.0
160	13	4.5

Exercise warmup routine

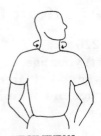

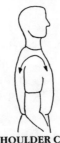

NECK TURNS
Turn head left to right, 4 times each side

SHOULDER CIRCLES
Both shoulders together frontwards and backwards 8 times each direction

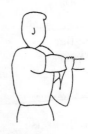

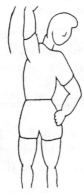

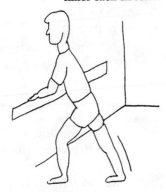

ARM STRETCH
Each arm for 8 counts

SIDE STRETCH
Hold each direction for 8 counts

CALF STRETCH
Hold each leg for 8 counts

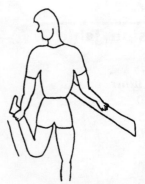

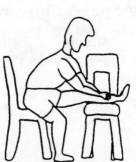

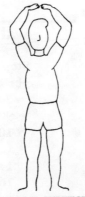

THIGH STRETCH
Hold each leg for 8 counts

HAMSTRING STRETCH
Hold each leg for 8 counts

FULL BODY STRETCH
Hold stance for 8 counts

Unfortunately, 50 percent of the people who start exercise programs drop out. We feel very lucky that only 36 percent of our patients dropped out in a three-year follow-up study. Out of this group of 36 percent, 40 percent of them dropped out because of time constraints. About the same number dropped out because it was boring. The rest had varied reasons.

Our patients choose to keep exercising for a very simple reason: They have chosen to take charge of their lives and they are determined not to let this deadly disease bother them again. On top of that, everybody is content and happy with the quality of their life, and that makes me happy.

Fat has twice as many calories as protein or carbohydrates, and the body easily converts calories from dietary fat to body fat. Using only 2.5 calories a day, our bodies can store 100 fat calories as body fat. For the same number of calories from protein or carbohydrate sources, the body spends 23 calories to store it as fat, almost ten times as much. Only 1 percent of protein and carbohydrates in our diet ends up as body fat because our bodies would rather use up those calories right away rather than spending ten times the energy it takes to store it.

Women should pay special attention to the following statistics:

If you are 5% overweight, your chance of developing coronary artery disease is 30% higher than it is for a woman of normal weight

If you are 15 to 20% overweight your chance of developing coronary artery disease is 80% higher than normal

If you are more than 30% overweight, your chance of developing coronary artery disease is 300% higher (three times more likely) than if your weight was normal.

Here's what you have to do to lose weight:

Step 1. Calculate your calorie needs for a moderately active lifestyle. (For a 120-pound woman it would be 1654 calories.)

Step 2. To lose one pound a week (a sensible and acceptable rate of weigh loss) you need to cut out 500 calories every day.

    i. One hour of exercise will burn 300 calories.

    ii. Cut only 200 calories from diet.

Why 500 calories? Because you need to burn 3500 calories to lose one pound of fat per week. By dividing 3500 by 7 days, you come up with 500 calories a day.

You can't lose weight unless you consume fewer calories than your body requires to carry out your daily activities. How many calories this is depends on your gender, age and activity level and is based on your Resting Metabolic Rate.

Daily Energy Requirement
(Owen's method)

Men

Resting Metabolic Rate = 10 x weight in pounds/2.2 + 900

Women

Resting Metabolic Rate = 7 x weight in pounds/2.2 + 800

For example, the Resting Metabolic Rate for a man weighing 150 pounds would be—

10 x 150/2.2 + 900 = 10 x 68 + 900 = 1,580 calories

For a woman weighing 120 pounds the Resting Metabolic Rate would be—

7 x 120/2.2 + 800 = 7 x 54.5 + 800 + 1,181.5 calories

Now multiply the Resting Metabolic Rate by the Activity Factor based on your total level of physical activity.

Low Activity = 1.2 Activity Factor

Moderate Activity = 1.4 Activity Factor

High Activity (athlete) = 1.6 Activity Factor

Most of us probably consider ourselves at a moderate activity level, so the amount of energy from calories that a man weighing 150 pounds would need to maintain his weight is—

1,580 (Resting Metabolic Rate) x 1.4 (Activity Factor) = 2,212 calories

A woman weighing 120 pounds will need—

1,181.5 (Resting Metabolic Rate) x 1.4 (Activity Factor) = 1,654 calories per day to maintain her weight.

10

Surya Namaskar Exercise

"Sun is the sustainer of the universe, comprised of movables and immovables."
Rig Veda:1,115-1

IN SANSKRIT SURYA MEANS "SUN," AND NAMASKAR means "bowing down." Sun is the powerhouse of the solar system. The radiant energy received from the sun is responsible for the existence of all living organisms on the earth. Surya Namaskar can be performed by all men and women;

This mode of ancient exercise is done to enhance the flexibility of the muscles and is a warmup exercise for everybody before the body is subjected to the abuse of everyday activity. Doing this exercise every morning will prime the muscles and ligaments with flexion and extension exercises. It is also a means of doing breathing exercises to breathe in fresh and clean morning air and increase the air exchange in the lungs which were sluggish during the sleep. It also stimulates the vagal nervous system to maintain the heart's pumping system.

This yogic exercise was developed in India thousands of years ago. There is no subtle philosophy or mysticism behind this nonsectarian mode of flexion and extension physical exercise.

When and how to practice Surya Namaskar

The Surya Namaskar exercise should be done early in the morning. Doing so helps invigorate the whole body by removing the stiffness in the body resulting from lying still all night. If possible it should be done after going to the toilet (hope so!) and should be done on an empty stomach. After the exercise allow the body to cool off before taking a shower.

Namaskar actually consists of a cycle of twelve progressive, connected positions. Perform the Namaskar slowly at your own pace, pausing for about five seconds, at each of the twelve positions. It is better to practice each one slowly and systematically with the appropriate breathing cycle rather than rushing through a large number of them.

No warmup exercises are needed to do the Namaskar as the routine itself is a sort of warming up exercise for the body. Initially do only one or two of this complete cycle of exercises. Later on you can increase slowly to perform for about fifteen minutes every day. If you are hurting while performing the Namaskar, then you are doing too much. The idea is to relax and loosen up the muscles so that the body can perform at the optimal level throughout the day. If you are hurting then it means the body, which was stiff and lazy because of the night's sleep, is working at the anaerobic level releasing lactic acid which is exactly what you do not want to do.

Breathing should be done rhythmically with the exercises. Coordinate the rhythm of the exercise with the rhythm of breathing. You will slowly learn how to do this along with the sequence of the movements. The breathing cycle will be easy if you remember that you should exhale as you bend forward and inhale when you are bending backward.

Namaskar

Sequentially Connected 12-Step Warmup Exercises

Begin this exercise in a standing position.

Step 1. Standing upright, touch both of your hands together, like a prayer hand, with the thumbs touching the groove in the middle of the top of the chest below your thyroid gland; exhale out as much as possible and hold for five seconds.

Step 2. Inhale and at the same time stretch your arms together in front and then vertically above your head and hold your breath. In the next five seconds while holding your breath, bend backwards as much as possible.

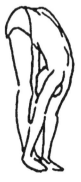

Step 3. Now double over and in this process exhale and hold your breath for five seconds.

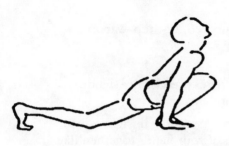

Step 4. Lift your left leg back while pressing down hard on the floor with the palm of your hands. While extending your left leg raise your trunk and head and inhale, holding your breath for five seconds.

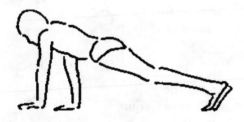

Step 5. While exhaling stretch only your right leg backward. Keep both legs straight.

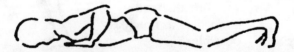

Step 6. Inhale and exhale slowly. While exhaling, bend elbows and knees and bring the body slowly to your knees, upper chest and forehead on the ground while keeping the lower abdomen, pelvis and thigh above the ground. Complete the exhalation holding your breath for five seconds.

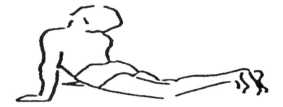

Step 7. Lower your pelvis to the floor. While you are inhaling, keep your hips touching the ground and raise your head first, then the upper and lower parts of the chest. Arch the spine as much as possible. Keep the knee touching the floor and look up at the sky or ceiling. Complete the inhalation and hold your breath for five seconds.

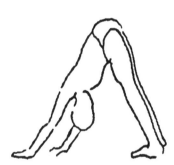

Step 8. Start exhaling slowly, pressing your hand and toes to the floor. Raise your knees slowly and lift your hips as high as possible. Arch your back and try to place your feet flat on the floor. Complete the exhalation and hold for five seconds.

Step 9. Inhaling slowly, bend your left leg slightly and slide your left foot behind your left arm. Bend your right knee and keep it a little above the floor. Raise your trunk and head. Thrust your chest forward and stretch your neck, chest and shoulders arching your spine to the maximum. Look up and complete the inhalation while holding your breath for five seconds.

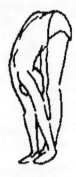

Step 10. While exhaling bend the right knee and slide the right foot forward up to the left foot. While doing so raise the hips keeping the palms touching the floor. Keep the head between the arms and complete the exhalation process.

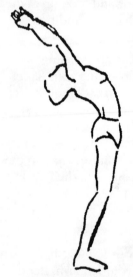

Step 11. While inhaling, stretch your arms and upper body slowly, rising up keeping your head between your arms and bringing your arms above your head. Complete the process of inhalation and hold your breath. Continuing to hold your breath, pull your arms backwards as much as possible.

Step 12. Now exhaling, bend forward and lower your arm slowly to the folding position in the middle of the chest and complete the exhalation. Bring your arm to your side and stand upright to start a new cycle.

Summary: 12-Step Surya Namaskar

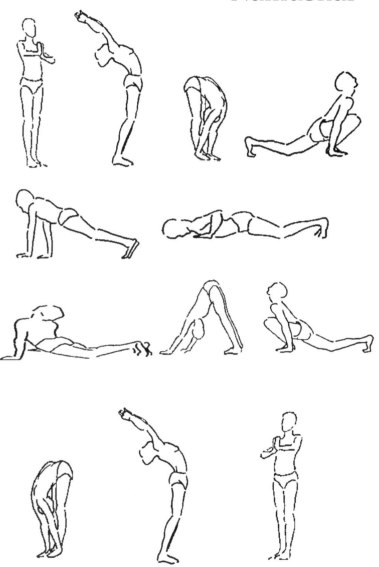

11

Eating Healthy

"Nature, time and patience—the best physicians."—Chinese fortune cookie.

WHILE MANY FACTORS CONTRIBUTE TO HEART disease, diet is one that most people recognize as being at least moderately controllable. We are living in an age that makes changing a little easier. Not too many years ago dietitians often started diet instruction for our patients with an apology: "I am sorry, but you will need to give up. . . eggs, cheese, ice cream, salad dressing, pies, cakes, cookies and on and on and on."

The very idea of starting a heart healthy diet was enough to make a person shake in his boots. But thanks to the response of many manufacturers to consumer needs we now have countless products to substitute for their previous high fat, artery clogging counterparts. And despite rumors to the contrary, we can actually like what we are eating while improving our cardiac health at the same time.

Some people who are overweight are distressed by their apparent inability to control their weight. Others do not seem to mind at all that they are overweight. Among all who are overweight exists a vast majority who have tried diet after diet, losing weight only to regain it.

Is being overweight actually harmful?

The answer is, Yes. And it is your heart that pays the highest price for every extra pound. For each extra pound of /body fat, the heart must pump blood through an extra *mile* of blood vessels. In addition to the physical burden on your heart, obesity increases the likelihood of developing atherosclerosis, high blood pressure, and diabetes. These conditions increase the risk of heart attack and stroke. The very nature of obesity leads to a more sedentary lifestyle. And a more sedentary lifestyle increases the risk of heart disease.

So what can be done to gain control of your weight and, as a consequence, your health? Two main causes of being overweight are an unbalanced diet and lack of exercise. Diets high in fat contribute to excessive calories and fatty deposits on the inside of arterial walls. A big first step in weight reduction and control lies in the selection and preparation of food. A trip to the grocery store is not the same as it was even ten years ago. It is impossible to shop without seeing products labeled "light," "low fat," "lowered fat," "reduced fat" and "nonfat."

With all the emphasis on eliminating or reducing the majority of fat from our diet, we should reach the conclusion that eating foods that contain too much fat is not good for us. We can hide from the truth and ignore dietary fats. But the truth is, too much dietary fat is harmful to our bodies, especially our hearts.

If you have ever looked on the label of any edible product, you will not be surprised to see the fat content listed first under nutrition facts. Cholesterol is normally listed after fats. Often fat will be subdivided into saturated and unsaturated, monounsaturated, and polyunsaturated. What does it all mean to the average person trying to eat healthy? Greater care needs to be taken in the selection of food since many foods can affect your blood lipid levels, especially your level of cholesterol and triglycerides.

Cholesterol is a fat-like substance derived from animal and dairy products. Cholesterol and triglycerides circulate in the bloodstream in complex substances known as lipoproteins. Lipoproteins are a combination of fat, *lipo*, and protein. Lipoproteins with small amounts of fat and cholesterol and large amounts of protein are referred to as high-density lipoproteins or HDL. This HDL cholesterol, or good cholesterol, removes cholesterol from the endothelium, or interior of the artery's walls.

Conversely, lipoproteins with large amounts of fat and cholesterol and small amounts of protein are known as low-density lipoproteins or LDL. We now know that too much cholesterol, especially the low density lipoprotein or LDL cholesterol, in our body can cause fatty deposits or plaque to build up in the interior walls of the coronary arteries. These fatty deposits or atheromas restrict blood flow and oxygen to the heart increasing the likelihood of heart disease, heart attack, and stroke.

Saturated fats remain solid at room temperature and are found mostly in animal and dairy products. Palm and coconut oils, two tropical oils, also are high in saturated fat, as are desserts made from them. Red meats, lard, butter, poultry with the skin left on, and whole milk dairy products are high in saturated fat. Saturated fats are linked to higher cholesterol levels which damage the heart and may also cause cancer.

Unsaturated fats are distinguished from saturated fats by their chemical composition. In unsaturated fats, there is room for additional hydrogen atoms to bond to the molecule; in saturated fats, the fat molecule is *saturated*, and there is no room for additional hydrogen atoms to bond to the molecule. Unsaturated fats are classified as monounsaturated, which means they bond two additional hydrogen atoms to the molecule, and polyunsaturated, which means they bond more than two hydrogen atoms.

Unsaturated fats, which remain liquid at room temperature, occur primarily in vegetable oils. Olive oil and peanut oil are types of monounsaturated fats; safflower, sunflower, soy, canola and corn oils are polyunsaturated fats. Unsaturated fats provide the body with linoleic acid which helps the body to absorb fat soluble vitamins. Linoleic acid is one of the few fatty acids that the body does not produce. One tablespoon of unsaturated fat daily will provide the body with enough fat to produce linoleic acid.

Omega-3 fatty acids, or fish oils prevalent in salmon, sardines, and mackerel, may help to lower cholesterol. Soluble fibers found in fruits such as apples and in vegetables such as broccoli, potatoes, and carrots help to lower cholesterol, in addition to legumes such as peas, beans, and lentils and whole grains such as oats and barley.

Cardiac rehabilitation patients at the Coronary Prevention and Rehabilitation Center limit their fat intake to twenty grams of fat daily. After reading about dietary fats, you may be wondering, "What can I eat?" There are many foods you can eat that are naturally low in cholesterol and fat. Your first plan of action should be to read labels at the grocery store. Pay attention to the number of fat grams per serving and check to see what the serving size is. Is it one half cup, three ounces, two tablespoons?

To trim fat calories naturally, buy foods which are low in fat: fresh fruits and vegetables, poultry without the skin, whole grain breads and cereals, fish, and lean cuts of meat marked "select." You can buy low fat or skim milk, nonfat yogurts, cheeses, and ice cream or cheeses made with part skim milk. Tub margarine is lower in fat than stick margarine. Watch out for baked goods which contain palm and coconut oils; nonfat baked goods are available.

When cooking, do not use additional fats. You can bake, broil, steam, poach, and microwave instead of frying and sautéing. Trim all visible fat off meats and avoid high fat processed meats like hot dogs and salami. You can use non-stick vegetable oils on grills and pans to prevent sticking. Use egg substitutes or egg whites in place of eggs, which are extremely high in cholesterol.

Use herbs instead of salt when seasoning; salt can cause blood pressure to rise. You can use fresh or dried herbs and experiment to see which ones you like. Nonfat yogurt and fat free mayonnaise and sour cream can be substituted for regular mayonnaise and sour cream in cooking and as toppings. In addition, lemon juice, lime juice, or vinegar are alternatives for high fat salad dressings. And watch your intake of sugar and hidden sugars which do not provide nutritional value but are high in calories.

Many snacks and cookies that are labeled as low fat or nonfat are high in calories, and the serving size is small. Sometimes people on low-fat or nonfat diets, have difficulty losing weight because they are eating at least as many calories as before. Often people have a tendency to think that they can eat more of an item that is labeled low fat or nonfat. You must read the label for calories and serving size.

Low fat does not mean no taste. People who are successful in reducing the majority of fats from their diet report that after about three weeks they do not miss eating high-fat foods. In addition to losing weight, they report that they feel better and look better as well. Developing a liking for certain foods is often the result of eating that food over a period of time. Since taste is acquired, you can add low fat foods that you enjoy to replace foods with a high fat content.

Finally you must read the food labels. I always recommend my patients to read only two things. One is fat content and the other is the number of calories in the food you are buying. Using the simple calculator printed on page 180 in this book you can easily calculate the percent of calories coming from fat in the particular item you are planning to buy. There are two rules of thumb that I follow. One, if the food I am buying has more than three grams of fat per serving then I will not buy it and will look for alternatives. The other is that I will buy food only if it has less then 30 percent of calories from fat. Using the calculator (which you could copy and keep in your wallet or purse) and after checking the fat and calories; you can calculate the amount of fat calories in the food you are buying.

Suppose in one of the examples the food item you are planning to purchase has eight grams of fat and 175 calories. If you draw the lines together on the calculator, the calories from fat in your food are 41 percent. I will not buy this food and will look for an alternative. If I could find the same item with six grams of fat and same number of calories I will buy it because now it has only 31 percent of calories coming from fat. Don't look for "zero" cholesterol advertised on the food box. This claim is printed to persuade you to buy the product, which may actually be weighted down with saturated fat.

Many cookbooks cater to low fat or nonfat cooking. The following recipes will allow you to try dishes that are healthy and taste good, too. These recipes were provided by our patients and tested by them and their spouses under the direction and guidance of our chief dietician, Liz Mount, R.D.

Every recipe was evaluated by her to make sure it is heart healthy, with substitutions as necessary. Then all of these recipes were cooked and tasted by her audience during our monthly Heart Healthy cooking demonstrations. All of these recipes are approved by us to be healthy, tasty and easy to prepare.

I am thankful to all who contributed recipes so that I could share them with a larger audience. I have tasted every one of them myself, and, believe me, you will love all of them.

After all, eating healthy is acquiring the habit of eating smart. Instead of trying to diet, which rarely works for people over a long period of time, you need to develop a new relationship to food, and eat healthier, low fat and nonfat foods. Start by incorporating a healthy, well-balanced assortment of foods into your meals that are naturally low in fat and learn to enjoy eating light. Where your heart is concerned, eating light is right thing to do.

BREAD, CAKE & COOKIES

Dill Bread

1 package active dry yeast
1/4 cup warm water
1 cup fat free cottage cheese
2 Tbs. sugar
1 Tbs. minced onion

2 1/2 cups all purpose flour
1 Tbs. low calorie margarine
2 tsp. dill seed
1 tsp. salt
1/4 tsp. baking soda
1 egg substitute

Dissolve yeast in water. In large bowl, mix all other ingredients and yeast mixture. Let the mixture rise for about one hour. Punch down. Place the mixture in pan and let it rise again about 45 minutes. Bake at 350 degrees for about an hour. Remove from the oven.

Yield: 15 slices

Nutrition information per slice:

Calories: 98 (11% from fat)
Carbohydrates: 16.8 gm
Fat: 1.24 gm
Sodium: 248 mg

Carrot Bread

1 1/3 cups sugar (or 3/4 cup
sugar plus 8 packets Equal)
1 1/3 cups *cold* water
1 cup raisins
1 tsp. cinnamon
1 tsp. nutmeg
3/4 tsp. ground cloves

2 Tbs. unsweetened
applesauce
3/4 cup cooked mashed
carrots
2 cups flour
2 tsp. baking soda
1/2 tsp. salt
1/2 cup walnuts, chopped

Combine the sugar, water, raisins, cinnamon, nutmeg, cloves, and applesauce in a saucepan and bring to a full boil over medium heat. Continue cooking for 5 minutes. Remove from heat and let stand till completely cooled. Add 3/4 cup cooked mashed carrots, blending well. Sift together flour, baking soda, and salt. Add this to the previous mixture. Add nuts, while mixing it well. Pour equally into 2 pans, 7 1/2 inches by 3 1/2 inches by 2 inches. Bake at 350 degrees for 1 hour. Let it cool down in pans about 5 minutes before removing.

Yield: 30 half-inch slices.

Nutrition information per half-inch slice:

Calories: 96 with all sugar (9% from fat),
   81 with sugar and Equal
Fat: 1 gm
Carbohydrate: 21 gm with all sugar,
   17 with sugar and Equal
Sodium: 95 mg

Cinnamon Coffee Cake

1 1/2 cups sifted flour
2 1/2 tsp. baking powder
1/2 cup sugar

1 egg white
1/4 cup unsweetened
   applesauce
3/4 cup skim milk

Sift together flour, baking powder, and sugar. Blend in egg
white, applesauce, and milk. Stir until flour is moistened.
Topping:

1/2 cup brown sugar
1/2 cup chopped pecans
   or walnuts (optional)

2 Tbs. flour
2 Tbs. oil
2 tsp. cinnamon

Make the topping by mixing together brown sugar, nuts, flour,
oil and cinnamon.
Spread half the batter in an oiled 8-inch square pan. Sprinkle
with half the topping. Add the remaining batter and sprinkle
with the rest of the topping. Bake at 375 degrees for 30
minutes or until done.
Yield: 9 servings.
Nutrition information per serving:
   Calories: 202 with no nuts (13% from fat)
   286 with nuts (35% from fat)
   Fat: 3 gm with no nuts, 11 gm with nuts
   Carbohydrates: 42 gm
   Sodium: 121 mg

Summer Cake

1 angel food cake
2 small packages sugar-
   free Jell-O
Fat-free whipped topping

2 cups fruit
2 small packages vanilla
   sugar-free pudding

Use any flavor Jell-O that will complement a fresh or canned
fruit (in unsweetened juice). i.e. strawberry Jell-O with fresh
strawberries, strawberry Jell-O with fresh bananas, peach Jell-O
with peaches, cherry Jell-O with cherries.

Tear up a whole angel food cake into small pieces. Arrange pieces in bottom of 13 x 9 inch pan. Set aside. In medium size bowl, empty packages of Jell-O. Add hot water- 1 cup per box as directed. Do not add cold water. Pour hot concentrated Jell-O onto angel food cake pieces in pan. Put in refrigerator and let it set. After Jell-O is set, cup up fresh fruit over cake. In medium size bowl, mix as directed: two small vanilla sugar free puddings (made with skim milk). Pour over fruit. Serve with fat free whipped topping on top (1 oz. per serving). Yield: 12 servings.

Nutrition information per serving:

Calories: 169 (0.5 % from fat)   Carbohydrates: 35.8 gm
Fat: 1.3 gm   Sodium: 402 mg

Quick Orange Streusel Cake

2 cups sifted flour	2 egg whites slightly beaten
1/2 cup sugar	1/2 cup skim milk
2 tsp. baking powder	1/2 cup orange juice
1 Tbs. grated orange rind	1/3 cup unsweetened applesauce

Sift together the flour, sugar and baking powder. Add the orange rind. Make a well in the dry ingredients and add the slightly beaten egg whites, milk, orange juice and applesauce. Stir until the mixture is dampened but still somewhat lumpy. Turn into a 10-inch pie pan or an 8 x 8 x 2-inch cake pan that has been sprayed with a non-stick coating.

Topping:

1/4 cup flour	2 Tbs. Margarine, reduced
1/2 cup sugar	fat

Mix the flour and sugar together then cut in the margarine to the consistency of cornmeal. Sprinkle over the cake batter and bake at 375 degrees for 35 minutes, or until browned.
Yield: 9 servings
Nutrition information per serving:

Calories: 241 (0.5% from fat)
Fat: 1.3 gm
Carbohydrates: 51 gm
Sodium: 127 mg

Oatmeal Cookies

3/4 cup applesauce
1/2 cup brown sugar
1/2 cup granulated sugar
2 egg whites
1/4 cup water
1 tsp. vanilla

1 cup flour
1/2 tsp. salt
1/2 tsp. baking soda
1 cup raisins
3 cups rolled oats, quick
   cooking or regular

Preheat oven to 350 degrees. Beat together applesauce, sugars, egg whites, water, and vanilla until creamy. Combine flour, salt, and soda. Add to creamed mixture. Add raisins and rolled oats. Mix well. Drop by rounded teaspoonfuls onto ungreased cookie sheet. Bake 12 to 15 minutes.

Yield: 5 dozen cookies

Nutrition information per cookie:

Calories: 124 (0% from fat)
Fat: 0 gm
Carbohydrates: 20 gm
Sodium: 47 mg

Almond Puffs

1 cup unsweetened applesauce
1 packet dry butter buds mix
1 cup sugar
1/4 cup egg substitute or
   2 egg whites

2 Tbs. almond extract
   (yes 2 Tbs.)
1 tsp. honey
3 cups flour
1 1/2 tsp. baking soda

Preheat oven to 350 degrees. Prepare cookie sheets with non-fat cooking spray. In a large mixer bowl blend applesauce and sugar. Add egg substitute, almond extract, vanilla and honey, beating until light and fluffy, scraping sides of bowl occasionally. Combine flour and baking soda; gradually add to creamed mixture until well blended. Drop dough by teaspoonful onto cookie sheets about 1 inch apart. Bake 7-8 minutes or until set.

Yield: 6 dozen cookies.

Nutrition information per cookie:

Calories: 30 (0% from fat)
Fat: 0 gm
Carbohydrate: 7 gm
Sodium: 17 mg

Rocky Road Brownies

4 egg whites	1/2 tsp. baking powder
1/2 cup sugar	1/2 tsp. salt
1 Tbs. vanilla	1/2 cup flour
1/2 cup cocoa powder	1 cup marshmallow creme

Preheat oven to 325 degrees. In a medium bowl, mix the egg whites with the next 6 ingredients adding each, one at a time, and beating well after each addition. Mix in the marshmallow creme just enough so it creates brown and white swirls. Spoon into a 9 by 13 inch pan that has been coated with a non-stick cooking spray. Bake for 18 minutes, 20 minutes for a more cake-like brownie. Cool and serve.
Yield: 15 brownies.
Nutrition information per serving:
        Calories: 150 (0% from fat)
        Fat: 0.5 gm
        Carbohydrate: 36 gm
        Sodium: 122 mg

SOUPS

Potato Cheddar Soup

4 cups peeled, cubed baking potato	2 Tbs. chopped fresh parsley
2 1/2 cups water	2 Tbs. chopped fresh chives
3/4 cup sliced carrot	1/8 tsp. salt
1/2 cup sliced celery	1/4 tsp. pepper
1/2 cup chopped onion	3/4 cup (3 oz.) shredded fat-free sharp Cheddar cheese
1 1/2 cup skim milk	Dash of hot sauce

Combine first 5 ingredients in a medium saucepan: bring to a boil. Reduce heat, and simmer, uncovered, 20 minutes or until vegetables are tender. Drain well, reserving 1 1/2 cups cooking liquid.Position knife blade in food processor bowl; add half of vegetable mixture and half of reserved cooking liquid. Process until smooth, and pour into saucepan. Repeat procedure with remaining vegetable mixture and reserved cooking liquid.
Add milk, chives, parsley, salt, and pepper to pureed vegetable mixture; cook over medium heat 5 minutes or until thor-

oughly heated, stirring occasionally. Add cheese and hot sauce, stirring until cheese softens.

Yield: 1 1/2 quarts (6, 1 cup servings)
Nutrition information per serving:
Calories: 164 (0% from fat)
Fat: 0 gm
Carbohydrates: 13.6 gm
Sodium: 183 mg

Chicken Mixed Vegetable Soup

3 1/2 cups water
1 Tbs. chicken-flavored bouillon granules (low sodium)
1 (14 1/2 oz.) can no-salt-added whole tomatoes, undrained and chopped
1/2 cup chopped fresh onion
1 tsp. dried whole basil
1 tsp. paprika
1 tsp. minced garlic
1/8 tsp. salt
1 cup sliced carrots
1 (8 oz.) can mushrooms stems and pieces, drained
1 cup diced zucchini
1 cup diced, cooked chicken

Combine water, bouillon granules, tomato, onion, basil, paprika, garlic, and salt in a Dutch oven. Bring to a boil; cover, reduce heat, and simmer 10 minutes. Add carrot; cover and simmer 10 minutes. Add mushrooms, zucchini, and chicken. Simmer, uncovered, 8 minutes.

Yield: 7 (1 cup) servings
Nutrition information per serving:
Calories: 82 (23% from fat)
Fat: 2.1 gm
Carbohydrates: 9.8 gm
Sodium: 429 mg

Tex-Mex Soup

3 1/2 cups canned low-sodium chicken broth, undiluted
1 cup chopped onion
1 cup chopped green pepper
1 cup chopped tomato
1/2 cup chopped fresh
parsley
1 tsp. dried while oregano
1 1/2 tsp. chili powder
1 tsp. ground cumin
1/8 tsp. salt
1/4 tsp. pepper
1 bay leaf

1 cup diced cooked chicken breast (skinned before cooking and cooked without salt)
2 Tbs. (1/2 oz.) shredded sharp fat free cheddar cheese

Light tortilla chips

Combine first 11 ingredients in a large saucepan, stirring well.
Bring to a boil; cover, reduce heat, and simmer 30 minutes,
stirring occasionally. Remove and discard bay leaf. Add
chicken, and cook until thoroughly heated. Ladle soup into
individual bowls; top evenly with cheese. Serve with light
baked tortilla chips.
Yield: 4 (1 cup) servings, served with 8 chips
Nutrition information per serving:
        Calories: 165 (17% from fat)
        Fat: 3.1 gm
        Carbohydrates: 17.9 gm
        Sodium: 249 mg

SALADS

Vegetable Dip/Creamy Caesar Salad Dressing

1/2 cup fat free Miracle Whip dressing	Parmesan cheese 2 Tbs. water
1/4 cup lemon juice	1 clove garlic, minced
1/4 cup plain nonfat yogurt	1/4 tsp. anchovy paste
2 Tbs. chopped fresh parsley	Fresh leaves oregano or
2 Tbs. grated fat-free	basil, minced (optional)

Combine all ingredients and whisk smooth. Store in refrigerator in covered container. This can be used as a fresh vegetable
dip or as a Caesar salad dressing over romaine lettuce, imita-
tion bacon bits, and croutons.
Yield: 1 1/4 cups or 20 1 Tbs. servings.
Nutrition information per 1 Tbs. serving:
        Calories: 15 (0% from fat)
        Fat: 0 gm
        Carbohydrates: less than 1 gram
        Sodium: 92 mg

Layered 24-Hour Salad

3 cups shredded iceberg
  lettuce or any combination
  of lettuce
	Salt and pepper to taste
	1 (8 oz.) can sliced water
	  chestnuts, drained

2 cups grated carrots	1/2 cup fat-free Parmesan

l stalk celery, diced
1 cup finely diced onions
2 cups non-fat mozzarella
  cheese (grated)
1 1/2 cups frozen Bird's
  Eye green peas

cheese
1 pint Kraft fat-free
  mayonnaise or Miracle
  Whip
1/2 cup fat-free sour cream

In a very large salad bowl line the bottom with bite-sized pieces of lettuce. Cover the lettuce with carrots, celery, onions, water chestnuts, and peas. Spread the pint of mayonnaise mixed with fat-free sour cream on top as if you are icing a cake. Sprinkle mozzarella and Parmesan cheese on top. Cover and refrigerate for 24 hours. Yields 16 servings.

Nutrition Information per serving:

Calories: 89
Fat: 0.1 gm (1% of calories from fat)
Cholesterol: 2 mg
Sodium: 675 mg
Carbohydrate: 19 g

Apple, Orange Slaw

2 cups shredded cabbage
1 small can mandarin oranges,
  drained
1 large red Delicious

apple, cored and diced
1/2 cup fat-free Miracle Whip
1 Tbs. brown sugar (or 1/4
  tsp. Sweet 'N Low Brown)

Place first three ingredients in a bowl, tossing to combine. Combine mayonnaise and brown sugar. Add this mixture to cabbage mixture and coat well. Cover and chill several hours or overnight.

Yield: 4 servings

Nutrition information per serving:

Calories: 90 (80 with Sweet 'N Low Brown)
Protein: 1 gm
Fat: 0.2 gm
Carbohydrate: 23 gm (20 gm with Sweet 'N Low
  Brown)
Sodium: 289 mg

Colorful Corn Salad

1 2/3 cups frozen whole kernel
  corn
1 (4 oz.) far diced pimiento,

1/4 cup chopped green
  onions
1 Tbs. sugar

drained   2 Tbs. cider vinegar
1/2 cup chopped green   1 tsp. celery seeds
  pepper   1 tsp. vegetable oil

Cook corn according to package directions, omitting salt.
Drain well, and let cool. Combine corn, pimiento, and remain-
ing ingredients in a medium bowl, stirring well. Cover and
chill salad at least 3 hours.
Yield: 4 servings.
Nutrition information per 1/2 cup serving:
        Calories: 78 (14% from fat)
        Fat: 1.3 gm
        Carbohydrate: 16.7 gm
        Fiber: 1.7 gm

Couscous Salad

1 cup plus 2 tablespoons fat-   cucumber
  free chicken broth   1/4 cup chopped fresh
parsley
3/4 cup couscous, uncooked   3 tablespoons balsamic
2 cups chopped, unpeeled   vinegar
  tomato   1 tablespoon Dijon mustard
1 cup chopped red bell pepper   1/2 teaspoon grated lemon
1/2 cup chopped celery   rind
1/2 cup chopped, unpeeled   1/4 teaspoon black pepper

Bring broth to a boil in a medium saucepan and stir in
couscous. Remove from heat and let stand, covered, for 5
minutes; fluff with a fork. Uncover and let cool 10 minutes.
Combine cooked couscous, tomato, and next 4 ingredients in
a large bowl and toss gently. Combine vinegar and next 3
ingredients in a small bowl and stir with a wire whisk. Add to
couscous mixture; toss to coat. Serve chilled or at room
temperature.
Yield: 6 servings, serving size 1 cup.
Nutrition information per serving:
        Calories: 100 (5% from fat)
        Fat: 0.6 gm (0.2 gm saturated fat)
        Sodium: 117 mg
        Cholesterol: 0 mg

Cranberry Salad

1 large package black cherry
    gelatin
2 cups boiling water
1 cup cold water
1, 12 oz. package cranberries

1 large orange
1/4 cup broken pecans
3/4 cup finely chopped celery
1 cup sugar

Mix gelatin and 2 cups boiling water, stirring until gelatin
dissolves. Add 1 cup cold water and chill in 13 by 9 inch pan.
Grind together the cranberries and orange. Add pecans, celery,
and sugar mixing well. Add to gelatin mixture and refrigerate
till set.
Yield: 18 servings.
Nutrition information per serving:
        Calories: 106 (19% from fat)
        Fat: 2.2 gm
        Carbohydrate: 22 gm
        Sodium: 22 mg

Fruit and Pasta Salad

1 medium orange
1/4 cup plain fat free yogurt
1 tsp. sugar
Dash salt

1/4 cup tiny bow tie pasta,
    cooked and drained
2 medium apples, cored
    and chopped
2 Tbs. sliced green onions

Finely shred enough orange peel to make 1/2 tsp.; set aside.
Remove the remaining peel from orange and section orange
over a bowl to catch juice. Measure 2 Tbs. of the juice.
In a medium mixing bowl stir together orange peel, the 2
Tbsp. juice, the yogurt, sugar, and salt. Mix well. Add cooked
pasta, chopped apples, and sliced green onions; toss to coat.
Gently stir in orange sections. Cover and chill for 2 to 24
hours.
Yield: 6 servings.
Nutrition information per serving:
        Calories: 76 (0% from fat)
        Fat: 0 gm
        Carbohydrates: 18 gm
        Sodium: 30 mg

Layered Fresh Vegetable Salad

3 cups shredded iceberg lettuce
1 cup fresh spinach, washed

salt and pepper to taste
2 cups non-fat cheddar

and well drained
2 cups grated carrots
1 stalk celery, diced
1 cup finely diced onions
1 1/2 cups frozen sweet green
  peas

cheese (grated)
1/2 cup fat-free Parmesan
  cheese
1 pint Kraft fat-free mayonnaise or Miracle Whip
1/2 cup fat-free sour cream

In a very large salad bowl line the bottom with bite-sized pieces of lettuce. Cover the lettuce with spinach, carrots, celery, onions, and peas. Spread the pint of mayonnaise mixed with fat-free sour cream evenly on top. Sprinkle cheddar and Parmesan cheeses on top. Cover and refrigerate for 24 hours. Yield: 16 servings.

Nutrition information per serving:
> Calories: 89 (1% from fat)
> Fat: 0.1 gm
> Cholesterol: 2 mg
> Carbohydrate: 19 gm
> Sodium: 675 mg

MAIN DISHES

Vegetarian Chili

1 stalk celery, chopped
1 large green pepper, chopped
1 large onion, chopped
2 cloves garlic, minced
3/4 cup bulgur
1 1/2 cup water
16 oz. V8 juice
2 Tbs. tomato paste

1/2 tsp. oregano
1/2 tsp. cumin
1 Tbs. chili powder
1 Tbs. soy sauce
  dash of tobasco sauce
15 oz. can kidney beans,
  drained and rinsed
1/2 cup frozen corn (de-
  frosted)

Sauté celery, green pepper, onion and garlic in Pam spray for two to three minutes. Add bulgur, tomato juice, tomato paste, spices, soy sauce, and tobasco sauce. Bring to a boil, cover and simmer on low for fifteen minutes. Add beans and corn. Cover and simmer for another 20 minutes. Yield: 10 servings.

Nutrition information per serving:
> Calories: 125 (0% from fat)
> Fat: 0 gm
> Carbohydrate: 14 gm
> Sodium: 430 mg

Grilled Vegetable Kabobs with Rice

1/2 cup commercial oil-free
Italian dressing
1 1/2 tsp. dried parsley flakes
1 1/2 tsp. dried whole basil
2 medium-sized yellow squash,
cut into 1-inch slices
2 medium-sized zucchini, cut
into 1-inch slices
8 small boiling onions
8 cherry tomatoes
8 medium-size fresh mush-
rooms
Vegetable cooking spray
2 cups cooked long-grain
rice (cooked without salt or
fat)

Combine dressing, parsley, and basil in a small bowl; cover and
chill. Alternate squash, zucchini, onions, tomatoes, and
mushrooms on 8 skewers. Coat grill rack with cooking spray;
place on grill over medium coals. Place kabobs on rack, and
cook 15 minutes or until vegetables are tender, turning and
basting frequently with dressing mixture. To serve, place 1/2
cup rice on each plate, and top with 2 vegetable kabobs.
Yield: 4 servings
Nutrition information per serving
        Calories: 184 (4% from fat)
        Fat: 0.8 gm
        Carbohydrates: 40 gm
        Sodium: 331 mg

Zingy Broccoli

1 (12 oz.) package frozen broccoli spears
1/4 cup fat-free Italian dressing

Arrange broccoli in a vegetable steamer over boiling water.
Cover and steam 8 minutes or until crisp-tender.
Place dressing in a 1-cup glass measure. Microwave at HIGH 1
minute or until hot, stirring after 30 seconds. Drizzle over
broccoli.
Yield: 4 servings.
Nutrition information per serving:
Calories: 36 (18% from fat)
        Fat: 0.7 gm (saturated fat 0.1 gm)
        Carbohydrate: 6.3 gm
        Cholesterol: 0 mg
        Sodium: 240 mg

Mexican Egg Casserole

4 corn tortillas, halved
1 cup chopped onion
1/4 cup chopped green pepper
1/4 cup chopped red pepper
1 tsp. minced garlic (in a jar)
1 tsp. ground oregano leaves
1 Tbs. parsley flakes
1/2 tsp. ground cumin
1 Tbs. fat-free chicken broth
2 cups canned kidney beans (rinsed and drained)
1 cup non-fat Cheddar cheese (grated)
1 1/2 cups skim milk
4 Egg Beaters (1 carton) (1 cup)
Taco sauce or salsa (optional)

Arrange the tortilla pieces in the bottom of a 12 x 8 x 2-inch casserole dish that has been sprayed with a non-fat cooking spray. Set aside. In a non-stick skillet over medium heat, cook onion, green pepper, red pepper, garlic, oregano, parsley, and cumin in chicken broth until tender. Stir in kidney beans. Spoon 1/2 of the mixture over the tortillas; repeat layers once. Sprinkle with cheese and set aside. In a bowl, combine milk and Egg Beaters; pour evenly over cheese. Bake at 350 F. for 30-40 minutes or until puffed and golden brown. Let stand 10 minutes before serving. Serve with taco sauce or salsa if desired.

Yield: 8 servings
Nutrition information per serving:
> Calories: 146 (6 % from fat)
> Fat: 1 gm
> Carbohydrates: 22 gm
> Sodium: 412 mg
> Fiber: 4 gm

Rice Pilaf

1 tsp. no-salt-added chicken broth
3/4 cup chopped onion
2 Tbs. slivered almonds
1 cup brown rice, uncooked
3/4 cup water
1/8 tsp. pepper
1 (13 3/4 oz.) can no-salt-added chicken broth
1 (2 1/2 oz.) jar sliced mushrooms, drained
1 (2 oz.) jar diced pimiento, drained

1. Heat broth in a medium saucepan over medium-high heat. Add onion and almonds; sauté 5 minutes or until onion is

tender and almonds are toasted.
2. Add rice; sauté 1 minute. Add water and remaining ingredients; bring to a boil. Cover, reduce heat, and simmer 30 minutes or until liquid is absorbed.
3. Remove from heat, and let stand, covered, for 5 minutes.
Yield: 4 servings.
Nutrition information per serving:
      Calories: 114 (23% from fat)
      Fat: 1.5 gm (Saturated fat 0.3 gm)
      Carbohydrate: 19 gm
      Cholesterol: 0 mg
      Sodium: 76 mg

Zucchini in Marinara Sauce

2 to 3 small washed unpeeled zucchini, cut into bite-sized pieces
2 Tbs. chopped onion
1 large clove grated garlic
1, 12 or 16 oz. can tomato sauce
1/2 tsp. basil
1/4 tsp. oregano
Dash black and/or red pepper to taste
dash rosemary powder
crushed leaves (optional)
1/4 tsp. fennel seed (optional)
1 to 2 tsp. sugar to taste (optional)

Spray non-stick coating onto large skillet and add onion and garlic. Brown briefly. Add zucchini and a little water. Cover and let simmer for a few minutes. Tossing gently add tomato sauce, basil, oregano, pepper, rosemary, fennel, and sugar if desired. Stir gently and cover. Simmer for 30 to 40 minutes or till tender but not mushy. May need to add a little water if gets too thick.
Yield: 6 servings.
Nutrition information per serving:
      Calories: 71 (0% from fat)
      Fat: 0 gm
      Carbohydrates: 16.7 gm
      Sodium: 253 mg (15 mg if using salt-free tomato sauce)

SEA FOOD DISHES

Oven Baked Catfish

1 cup fine, dry bread crumbs	8 (6 oz.) dressed catfish
1 tsp. dried parsley	vegetable cooking spray
1 tsp. dried basil	lemon wedges (optional)
1/3 cup fat-free mayonnaise	Fresh parsley sprigs
1 1/2 Tbsp. water	(optional)

Lightly toss bread crumbs with dried parsley and basil. Place in shallow bowl. Combine mayonnaise and water stirring well. Dip fish in mayonnaise mixture then dredge in breadcrumb mixture. Place fish on a baking sheet coated with cooking spray. Bake at 450 degrees for 15 to 17 minutes or until fish flakes easily when tested with a fork. If desired, garnish with lemon wedges and fresh parsley sprigs.

Yield: 8 servings

Nutrition information per serving:
  Calories: 197 (24% from fat)
  Fat: 5.2 gm
  Carbohydrates: 13.3 gm
  Sodium: 298 mg

Orange and Saucy Orange Roughy

1 lb. orange roughy	1/2 tsp. paprika
1/4 cup frozen orange juice	1 Tbs. dried parsley
concentrate	1/2 cup water
2 Tbs. lemon juice	6 Tbs. orange marmalade,
1 1/2 tsp. dried dill weed	sweetened with fruit juice
	2 tsp. cornstarch

Spray non-metal casserole with vegetable cooking spray and place fish in casserole. Combine remaining ingredients except cornstarch stirring well. Pour over fish and marinate for 1 hour in refrigerator. Turn after about 1/2 hour. Preheat broiler. Remove fish from marinade, reserving marinade, and place fish on broiler pan. Broil fish 4 inches from heat 10-15 minutes, until fish flakes. Baste with marinade several times during cooking to keep moist. Heat rest of marinade in small saucepan with cornstarch until sauce begins to thicken. Serve fish with sauce and garnish with fresh orange slices if desired.

Yield: 4 servings

Nutrition information:

Calories: 163 (5% from fat)
Fat: 1 gram
Carbohydrates: 6 gm
Sodium: 99 mg

Salmon Crab Croquettes

8 oz. salmon fillet
8 oz. crab meat or substitute
2 tsp. mustard (Dijon)
2 Tbs. green onion (use only
  the green tops, chop finely)
Cracker crumbs (fat free)

1/2 sleeve finely ground
White pepper, to taste
Tabasco, to taste
1 tsp. Worcestershire sauce
1 egg white
Juice from 1/2 fresh lemon

Blanche salmon about three minutes in boiling water. Drain
thoroughly. Put in freezer a few minutes to cool. Check to
remove any possible bones. Combine remaining ingredients
except cracker crumbs. Toss with salmon and crab meat until
well blended. Divide into 6 patties and roll in cracker crumbs.
Brown in nonstick pan sprayed with Pam. Finish heating in
350 degree oven for about ten minutes or until heated
through. Serve with favorite sauce.
Yield: 6 servings.
Nutrition information per serving:
Calories: 107 (25% from fat)
Fat: 3 gm
Carbohydrates: 6 gm
Sodium: 375 mg

Orange Snapper

6 (4 oz.) red snapper fillets
  (1/2 inch thick)
Vegetable cooking spray
31/2 Tbs. water
2 Tbs. frozen orange juice
concentrate, thawed and

undiluted
1/2 tsp. grated orange rind
1/4 tsp. ground nutmeg
Dash of freshly ground
  pepper
Orange wedges (optional)

Arrange fillets in a 13 x 9 x 2-inch baking dish coated with
cooking spray. Combine water and next 4 ingredients; pour
over fillets. Bake, uncovered, at 350 degrees for 20 minutes or
until fish flakes easily when tested with a fork. When serving,
garnish with orange wedges if desired.
Yield: 6 servings

Nutrition information per serving:
Calories: 118 (11 % from fat)
Fat: 1.4 gm
Carbohydrates: 2.3 gm
Sodium: 49 mg

Shrimp Scampi

2 lbs. large raw shrimp
1/2 cup liquid Butter Buds
8 cloves garlic, crushed

1/3 cup chopped parsley
2 tsp. grated lemon peel
2 Tbs. lemon juice
1 lemon cut into 6 wedges

Preheat oven to 400 degrees. Peel and devein shrimp. Spray a
13 x 9 x 2-inch baking dish with a vegetable cooking spray.
Blend together liquid Butter Buds, garlic and 1/2 the parsley.
Pour into prepared dish. Arrange shrimp in single layer over
Butter Buds sauce. Bake uncovered, 5 minutes. Turn shrimp.
Sprinkle with lemon peel, lemon juice, and remaining parsley.
Bake 8-10 minutes longer or until just tender. Serve with rice.
Pour Butter Buds mixture over shrimp. You may garnish with
lemon wedges if you wish. If you use smaller shrimp cut back
on the cooking time as they get tough if over cooked.
Yield: 8 servings
Nutrition information per serving:
Calories: 264 (8% from fat)
Fat: 2.3 gm
Carbohydrate: 32 gm (with 1/2 cup cooked rice)
Sodium: 281 mg

POULTRY DISHES

Chicken Fajitas

4 (8 inch) flour tortillas
vegetable cooking spray
1 pound chicken breast
   tenders
1 tsp. chili powder
1/2 teaspoon ground cumin
1/2 tsp. pepper
1 Tbs. lime juice

2/3 cup sliced green onions
1/4 cup chopped fresh
   cilantro
1/2 cup plain nonfat yogurt
4 leaf lettuce leaves
8 (1/8 inch thick) slices
   unpeeled tomato, each cut
   in half crosswise

Wrap tortillas in damp paper towels and then in aluminum
foil. Bake at 350 degrees for 7 minutes or until softened; set
aside. Coat a large nonstick skillet with cooking spray; place

over medium-high heat until hot. Add chicken, chili powder, and cumin; saute 5 minutes or until chicken is done. Combine chicken, pepper, and lime juice in a bowl, and toss well. Add green onions, cilantro, and yogurt, and toss well. Place a lettuce leaf on each tortilla; divide chicken mixture evenly over lettuce. Top each with 4 tomato pieces; roll up.
Yield: 4 servings.
Nutrition information per serving:
  Calories: 290 (15% from fat)
  Fat: 4.8 gm.
  Carbohydrate: 28.3 gm

Chicken and Broccoli With Wild Rice

1 package (6 oz.) long-grain and wild rice
2 Tbs. cornstarch
1 cup skim milk
3/4 cup water
1/2 tsp. chicken flavored bouillon granules
Vegetable cooking spray
1/2 cup fresh mushrooms, cleaned and sliced
2 packages (10 oz. each)
frozen broccoli in spears or chopped, defrosted and drained
4 cups cooked chicken breasts, coarsely chopped and skinless
1/3 cup green onions, ends removed, sliced
1/4 cup bread crumbs
1/4 cup plus 2 tablespoons fat-free Parmesan cheese
2 tablespoons parsley

Cook rice according to package directions, omitting fat; set aside. This will take about 25 minutes. Preheat oven to 350 degrees. Mix cornstarch with skim milk, stirring until smooth in small saucepan. Cook over medium heat, stirring constantly until thickened and bubbly. Add water and bouillon granules, stirring until dissolved. Coat a small skillet with vegetable spray; place over medium heat until hot. Add mushrooms and onions and sauté two to three minutes or until tender. Stir rice, mushrooms and onions into cornstarch-milk mixture in saucepan. Coat a 9 x 13 inch baking dish lightly with cooking spray. Arrange broccoli on bottom. Top with chicken. Pour rice-mushroom-onion sauce over chicken. Sprinkle with bread crumbs, Parmesan cheese and parsley. Bake uncovered for thirty minutes or until top is golden brown.
Yield: 8 servings.

Nutrition information per serving:
>   Calories: 272
>   Fat: 6 gm (1 gm from saturated fat)
>   Carbohydrate: 29 gm
>   Sodium: 183 mg

Chicken Breasts Dijonnaise

1/4 cup fine, dry bread
  crumbs
1 Tbs. grated Parmesan
  cheese
1/2 tsp. dried whole thyme
1 tsp. basil

1/4 tsp. pepper
2 Tbs. creamy mustard-
  Dijonnaise
4 (3 oz.) skinned, boned
  chicken breast halves
vegetable cooking spray

1. Combine first 5 ingredients in a shallow dish; stir well, and set aside.
2. Brush mustard blend evenly over both sides of chicken. Dredge chicken in breadcrumb mixture.
3. Place chicken on a rack coated with cooking spray; place rack in shallow roasting pan. Bake at 375 for 45 minutes or until done.
Yield: 4 servings.
Nutrition information per serving:
>   Calories: 174 (14% from fat)
>   Fat: 2.8 gm (saturated fat 0.7 gm)
>   Carbohydrate: 6.8 gm
>   Cholesterol: 67 mg
>   Sodium: 381 mg

Hearty Lasagna

3/4 pound ground skinless
chicken breast
Vegetable cooking spray
1 cup chopped onion
3 garlic cloves, minced
1/4 cup chopped fresh
parsley, divided
1 (28-ounce) can whole
tomatoes, undrained and
chopped
1 (14 1/2-ounce) can Italian-
style stewed tomatoes,
undrained and chopped

tomato paste
2 teaspoons dried oregano
1 teaspoon dried basil
1/4 teaspoon pepper
2 cups nonfat cottage cheese
1/2 cup (1 ounce) fat-free
Parmesan cheese
1 (15-ounce) container
nonfat ricotta cheese
1 egg white, lightly beaten
12 cooked lasagna noodles
2 cups (8 ounce) shredded
fat-free mozzarella cheese

1 (8-ounce) can no-salt-
added tomato sauce
1 (6-ounce) can

fresh oregano sprigs
(optional)

Cook ground chicken in a large saucepan over medium heat until browned, stirring to crumble; drain and set aside. Wipe pan with a paper towel. Coat pan with cooking spray; add the onion and garlic, and sauté 5 minutes. Return chicken to pan. Add 2 tablespoons parsley and next 7 ingredients; bring to a boil. Cover, reduce heat, and simmer 15 minutes. Remove from heat. Combine remaining 2 tablespoons parsley, cottage cheese, and next 3 ingredients in a bowl; stir well, and set aside. Spread 3/4 cup tomato mixture in bottom of a 13 x 9-inch baking dish coated with cooking spray. Arrange 4 noodles over tomato mixture; top with half of cottage cheese mixture, 2 1/4 cups tomato mixture, and 2/3 cup mozzarella. Repeat layers, ending with noodles. Spread the remaining tomato mixture over noodles. Cover; bake at 350 for 1 hour. Sprinkle with remaining mozzarella; bake, uncovered for 10 minutes. Let stand 10 minutes before serving. Garnish with oregano, if desired.

Yield: 9 servings.

Nutrition information per serving:
   Calories: 380, 20% from fat
   Protein: 33.4 gm
   Fat: 8.5 gm
   Carbohydrates: 40.5 gm
   Sodium: 703 mg

Lime-Sauced Chicken

Nonstick spray coating
4 medium (12 oz. total)
   boned and skinless
   chicken breast halves
1/2 medium lime

3/4 cup apple juice or
   apple cider
2 tsp. cornstarch
1/2 tsp. instant chicken
   bouillon granules

Spray a large skillet with nonstick spray coating. Preheat skillet over medium heat. Add chicken. Cook over medium heat for 8 to 10 minutes or till tender and no longer pink, turning to brown evenly. Remove from skillet; keep warm. Meanwhile, remove strips of peel from lime, using a vegetable peeler. Cut peel into thin strips; set aside. Squeeze 1 Tbs. juice from lime. Combine lime juice, apple juice, cornstarch, and bouillon granules; carefully add to skillet. Cook and stir till

thickened and bubbly. Cook and stir 2 minutes more.
To serve, cut each chicken breast half into 1-inch diagonal
pieces. Spoon some sauce over each serving. Garnish with
reserved lime peel. Pass remaining sauce.
Yield: 4 servings.
Nutrition information per serving:

> Calories: 270 (10% from fat)
> Fat: 3 gm
> Carbohydrate: 7 gm
> Sodium: 111 mg
> Cholesterol: 72 mg

DESSERTS

Fruity Yogurt Ice

1, 15 or 16 oz. can red raspberries, peach slices, blueberries or apricots	28 oz. carton vanilla fat-free yogurt 1 Tbs. honey

Place undrained fruit in a blender container or food processor
bowl. Blend or process till smooth. If using raspberries, strain
them to remove seeds. In a medium mixing bowl stir together
blended fruit, yogurt, and honey. Pour into an 8x8x2-inch
pan. Cover and freeze for 3 to 4 hours or till firm. Break
frozen mixture into chunks with a wooden spoon and place in
a chilled large mixer bowl. Beat with an electric mixer on
medium speed till fluffy. Return to pan. Cover and freeze for 6
hours more or till firm. To serve, let mixture stand at room
temperature for 5 minutes; then scoop into dessert dishes.
Yield: 8 servings.
Nutrition information per serving:

> Calories: 108 (0% from fat)
> Fat: 0 gm
> Carbohydrates: 24 gm
> Sodium: 38 mg

Cranberry Crunch

1 cup uncooked rolled oats	1/8 tsp. salt
1/2 cup all purpose flour	1 egg white
2/3 cup brown sugar	2 Tbs. light corn syrup
1/4 tsp. baking powder	16 oz. can whole berry
1/4 tsp. cinnamon	cranberry sauce

Preheat oven to 350 degrees. Lightly spray an 8 x 8 inch baking pan with a non-stick coating spray. Combine oats, flour, brown sugar, baking powder, cinnamon and salt. Stir together egg white and corn syrup. Drizzle egg mixture over oat mixture, stirring and tossing gently with a fork until all ingredients are moist. Mixture will be crumbly. Press just over half into the bottom of the pan. Stir the cranberry sauce to break up chunks. Spoon cranberry sauce over mixture in pan. Sprinkle remaining oat mixture over cranberry sauce. Bake 40 to 45 minutes, until evenly browned on top. Serve warm or cool, plain or with a scoop of vanilla nonfat frozen dessert.
Yield: 9 servings.
Nutrition information per serving:
>   Calories: 230 (0% from fat)
>   Fat: 0.7 gm
>   Carbohydrates: 26 gm
>   Sodium: 46 mg

Blenderized Fruit Smoothie

1 can pineapple tidbits
   or chunks in own juice,
   no sugar added
2 large bananas, cut up
   in chunks

1 1/2 cups skim milk
3 packets Equal or
   Sweet 'N Low
5 ice cubes

Put all ingredients in blender and blend until smooth. Serve chilled.
Yield: 6 1-cup servings.
Nutrition information per serving:
>   Calories: 120
>   Carbohydrates: 30 gm
>   Fat: Trace
>   Sodium: 65 mg

FAT AND OIL—A PRAGMATIC APPROACH

What type of oil should I use?

Debate continues over the type of oil which is heart healthy. Many people think that a clear, golden-colored oil is inherently superior because of the clarity of the oil. People also have changed from using lard and butter to using highly refined polyunsaturated vegetable oils which are low in saturated fat. The intention is to prevent atherosclerosis, heart attack and stroke. But are we doing the right thing?

Margarine and shortening contain hydrogenated polyunsaturated vegetable oil which, through the process of hydrogenation, creates a type of synthetic fat that are known as trans fatty acids. Most margarines are actually made from soybean and sunflower oil and though sold as "natural" are also hydrogenated and are therefore harmful. Trans fatty acid is created when oils are partially hydrogenated so that the oil can be reused in deep frying. It also makes the crust crispier. To avoid eating trans fatty acid:

1. **Avoid deep-fried foods**
2. **Use tub margarine rather than sticks**
3. **Look for saturated or fat-free foods**
4. **Use olive and canola oil**

Clarified butter contains butyric acid which is supposed to be an antioxidant and also has anti cancer properties. It has been touted in Aurvedic literature to be antiviral, to increase the metabolism and to possibly prevent Alzheimer's Disease, although no scientific research has been done to demonstrate those properties.

What are the differences between refined and unrefined oil?

Unrefined oil is mechanically pressed under a relatively low temperature of less than 100 degrees, retaining the original taste and color. It also contains Vitamin E, which preserves the oil from rancidity and reduces free radical damage in the body that results from consumption of the polyunsaturated portion of the oil.

Refined oil is processed in a refinery at a relatively high temperature which exceeds 450 degrees. After World War II, an extraction method was developed to produce more oil at a cheaper price. This technique of extraction of oil by solvents has not changed for the last fifty years. After the seed is rolled and heated at about 150 degrees, Hexane, a chemical, is added as a solvent to extract the oil completely from the seeds. Then this solvent is evaporated at a temperature of about 300 degrees and is reused.

After this process the oil is degummed, and protein carbohydrate and many trace minerals and lecithin are removed. Sodium hydroxide is then added, removing linoleic acid and linolenic acid, two essential fatty acids which the body cannot produce. (By the way, sodium hydroxide is an active ingredient in Drano.) Under heat, the oil is bleached to make it transparent. Next the process of deodirization is performed to get rid of the horrible taste and smell that develop during the extraction process. This is done by distilling the oil at 500 degrees. The natural fatty acid (cis-fatty acid) is transformed into trans fatty acid. This is the same type of fatty acid that is formed during the hydrogenation while making margarine and shortening.. Because of this process, refined oil is depleted of the natural antioxidants which your body needs: lecithin, vitamin E, beta carotene, calcium, magnesium. At such a high temperature the unsaturated fatty acids change into synthetic fat known as trans fatty acids. (Trans fatty acid formation starts at about 320 degrees.) Trans Fatty acids may actually be worse for our health than saturated fat.

Although quite a bit of research has been done on trans fatty acids, not much has been published in lay literature. Scientists and industrial firms are working on creating a trans fatty acid free margarine which should be available to the general public soon. Solid margarine is full of trans fatty acids, while tub margarine or liquid margarine does not have such a quantity of trans fatty acids. In the USA 95 percent of trans fatty acids come into the typical diet from margarine and shortening.

Any time you use oil for cooking at a temperature above 320 degrees, the process of hydrogenation begins, changing the oil into trans fatty acids. Unfortunately, trans fatty acids increase cholesterol. The best way to avoid trans fatty acid is to avoid fried foods and high-fat bakery goods that contain hydrogenated and partially hydrogenated oils.

We know that fat is an important dietary constituent for our body. It provides us with energy and helps us move fat-soluble vitamins across the cell membranes and into the blood stream. We are still debating and it remains too close to call whether the oil which is predominately made of monounsaturated fat is better than polyunsaturated fat or vice versa.

One thing we know is that all oil is 100 percent fat. "Fat is a fat is a fat." However, it is extremely important to use oil which is stable. Some of the oils (such as safflower oil) are not stable at high temperatures and are not recommended for deep frying or stir frying. This type of oil is very unstable and is oxidized easily. Linoleic acid from the oil breaks down. If the oil is then left on the shelf too long, the linoleic acid is also oxidized and becomes rancid and toxic.

Oil high in monounsaturated fat has more oleic acid and less of the fatty acid such as linolenic acid and linoleic acid. This type of oil will break down easily. If the oil can or bottle has been opened, you must store it in darkness or in the refrigerator; otherwise it will become rancid.

Olive oil is the best oil to use. But it is important to know which olive oil is the best for our health. We know that the Mediterranean diet uses a lot of olive oil and that seems to be statistically helpful. However, that beneficial effect will vanish if you started using a refined and rancid olive oil.

Olive oil harvested earlier in the season has a fruitier taste and is a slightly green color. Oil harvested later in the season has a sharper, nuttier taste and is golden in color.

Extravirgin oil is extracted from top grade olives which were picked and quickly pressed without any heat and under a temperature of 100 degrees without adding any solvent. This process is called *cold pressed*, which means pressed at room temperature, and has a very low acid level.

The olive oil which does not qualify as extravirgin is refined chemically to lower the level of the acid. This oil is tasteless, odorless, lacks Vitamin E and is not considered heart healthy. Some companies add extra vitamin E to this *refined oil* to compensate for the loss of vitamin E, but there is nothing better than natural vitamin E.

Saturated Fat

Saturated fat is a cholesterol booster that will stimulate the liver to produce more cholesterol. It is made up of stearic acid and palmetic acid. The stearic acid which makes half of the saturated fat actually does not increase cholesterol. It is only the palmetic acid which increases cholesterol.

Unsaturated Fat

The unsaturated fats are not cholesterol boosters. There are three types.

1. Monounsaturated fat such as canola oil, olive oil, peanut oil and sesame oil.

2. Polyunsaturated fat (Omega 6) which is a corn oil.

3. Monounsaturated fat (Omega 3), fish oil. Omega 3 polyunsaturated fat may actually decrease heart disease as well as the risk of it and also interfere with blood clot formation.

Effects of oil on cholesterol

1. Saturated fatty acid will increase LDL.

2. Polyunsaturated fat decreases cholesterol, but decreases HDL also.

3. Monounsaturated fat has a neutral effect on cholesterol but will decrease LDL.

You should replace saturated fat by polyunsaturated or monounsaturated fat to decrease your total cholesterol and LDL-cholesterol. The word of wisdom is to use unrefined oil and use it in moderation. If you do that, then you will not go wrong even if you use monounsaturated fat or polyunsaturated fat.

It is important to know that if you are not eating too much fat but are consuming too many calories from carbohydrates and at the same time not exercising enough to take care of this excessive input of calories, this could be the source of your heart problems, too. Extra calories from carbohydrates will be converted into and stored as fat in your body.

If you eat food heavy in saturated fats but exercise quite a bit, while a friend of yours is not exercising at all and is eating a low-fat but high-calorie carbohydrate diet, which one of you is being kinder to your heart? Interestingly, your friend is accumulating more fatty acids in his or her body than you are, even though you are consuming a high saturated-fat diet but exercising more. The difference is that even with a high-fat diet and exercise you are burning off as many calories as you are consuming. The intake of the calories in any form should be neutralized by the output.

To learn more about the biochemical conversion of carbohydrates to saturated fat, the process of changing calories to fat, consult your local librarian for books on this topic.

All polyunsaturated vegetable oils (unless they are cold pressed) are heated during processing and are virtually a storehouse for free radicals.

Essential Fatty Acids

There are two families of essential fatty acids. One is *linoleic acid* and the other is *linolenic acid*. These essential fatty acids have three functions.

The most important function of these fatty acids is to form your cellular membranes. If you do not have enough of these fatty acids, the membranes of your cells will be faulty. We have trillions of cells in our body and because of natural wear and tear you need a constant supply of fatty acids to repair and create new cells.

Secondly, these acids help transport cholesterol.

Finally, they function as a precursors of the prostaglandins, which are formed only from essential fatty acids.

My recommendations for using oils are as follows:

a. **Oil for baking**

> **Monounsaturated oil such as canola oil or olive oil**
> **These oils have a tendency to lower bad cholesterol.**

b. **Oil for cooking**

> **Extra virgin olive oil**

c. **Oil for frying**

> **I hate to even recommend oil for deep frying, but if you must deep-fry foods, use either canola oil or high-oleic safflower oil. Use the oil only once and then discard it. Otherwise you will have trans fatty acids to deal with. You may want to add fresh garlic clove or onion to the oil while frying. This has been shown to work as an antioxident and retard the breakdown of the oil.**

In the 1930s cardiovascular disease was responsible for only fifteen percent of all the deaths in the US. Today it accounts for fifty percent of all deaths. In the 1930s only three percent of the US population was dying from cancer but now twenty-five percent of them are dying from cancer. Where did we go wrong? We thought that by using margarine rather than lard would take care of heart disease, but somehow that equation is not working to our advantage. It is possible that if we had not changed to margarine even more people would have died from heart disease. We'll never know. I firmly believe that it is not the oil which the sole cause of heart disease, but the lack of exercise and unmanageable stress in our post World War II era which is the main culprit.

Antioxidants

To understand antioxidants, it is important to understand the concept of free radicals. Free radicals are small molecules with an extra electron that is generated by the cells in the body upon exposure to toxins. This extra unpaired electron makes the molecule unstable because it lacks one of its electrons. It is released by the cells for its defense to destroy unwanted invaders by oxidation.

There seems to be a mini war being waged by trillions of cells in our body at their mini level to protect us from diseases. Come to think of it, they are fighting for our life. It is just like *Star Wars* with destructive forces being defeated by radicals released by brave cells. It is a humbling thought to see how meticulously our body is built to handle all these mini catastrophes. When cells can no longer fight the invasion of destructive and toxic forces, they themselves are attacked by the same free radicals they released to fight the invaders. This can cause cancer, heart disease and aging.

When an unstable molecule seeks to replace its missing electron, it causes a chain reaction that can cause damage to cell membranes and the cell's DNA. If these cells are unprotected, the free radicals disturb the action of cellular DNA; this in turn, disables them, possibly rendering them the foundation for cancer and other chronic diseases.

These free radicals are unavoidable; they are formed constantly in our body as a by-product of the normal consequence of metabolism. They are also derived from other sources such as air pollution, cigarettes, pesticides, chemicals, physical injury, exercise and emotional stress. The other source of free radicals is ischemia, when the blood supply to the cells is cut off as in obstructive coronary artery disease.

Free radicals are not all bad; they do improve the immune system. Our body produces them because they are needed for destroying unwanted invaders in our body. However after producing free radicals for their own protection, the cells themselves may also become targets and must ward off continuous unchecked bombardment of these radicals with an Antioxidant Defense Scavenger System (ADS System) composed of nutrients known as free radical scavengers.

These scavenger nutrients are bound up and metabolized by the ADS System consisting of antioxidants such as Vitamins A, C, E, the mineral selenium and bioflavanoids. If you are not exposed to unnecessary toxins, your body has enough of this ADS System provided by natural foods to protect yourself. But if you are exposed to these free radicals, it is a good idea to take antioxidant supplements.

Free radicals can change the LDL (bad cholesterol) to the more harmful form of oxidized bad cholesterol which can plug up the arteries. We know that this oxidation process causes chronic diseases, but does that mean that taking antioxidants can counteract or stop this progress? Fortunately, the body has a weapon to keep free radicals under control. Known as natural antioxidants, these molecules prevent and repair free radical damage and also clean up unstable molecules and get them out of the system.

The most important of the antioxidant enzymes in our bodies are catalase, superoxide dismutase and glutathione peroxidase. Supplemental antioxidants that you can take are Vitamin C, Vitamin E and beta carotene. We are still trying to find out if these antioxidants from outside will be of any help or not. The Monica study in Italy, France and Spain, and a few other countries showed that people consuming more fresh fruits and vegetables had a lower incidence of cardiovascular disease compared to people in countries such as Sweden where fewer fresh fruits and vegetables are available. Japan has a higher incidence of breast cancer compared to the United States, but colon cancer is higher in the US than in Japan. Is this difference caused by chemical toxins, use of preservatives or the effect of antioxidants? Several studies also show that low blood levels of antioxidants like vitamin C and E are associated with increased risk of heart disease.

Theoretically, it is possible to get all of the Vitamin B and C you need in your diet if you eat seven to nine servings of fruit and vegetables a day and prepare that with minimal cutting, peeling, trimming and cooking. However, Americans simply will not eat that many fruits and vegetables. I really feel that particularly, in the case of Vitamin E, which is found in fatty foods like nuts and seeds, it is impossible to get enough vitamin through the diet alone. The damaged and oxidized LDL cholesterol appears to accelerate atherogenesis and Vitamin E is thought to have an antioxidant property which will repair the damaged LDL cholesterol.

Researchers are still trying to design a diet rich in vitamins, fruits and vegetables, and particularly in greens, like cabbage and broccoli, to reduce the low incidence of cancer and other diseases.

The compound coenzyme Q-10, as well as the mineral selenium are thought to help neutralize the free radicals. However, this relationship has not been studied extensively. Too much selenium can cause fatigue and other severe toxic effects. Heavy drinkers should not take beta carotene at all and people who are on anticoagulants, such as Coumadin, should avoid taking Vitamin E because it can cause excessive bleeding. People with kidney stones should avoid taking Vitamin C. A nurse health study following 87,245 female nurses for eight years showed that nurses consuming higher beta carotene had 22 percent lower risk of coronary artery disease, and nurses consuming higher Vitamin E had 34 percent lower incidence of coronary artery disease.

A "health profession" study followed 39,910 members of the medical profession for three years. People taking higher beta carotene had a 25 percent lower incidence of coronary artery disease, and people consuming higher vitamin E experienced a 39 percent lower rate of coronary disease. "HOPE," or Heart Outcome Prevention Evaluation, was being conducted in nineteen countries in 1996 as this book is being prepared for printing. The study is checking the role of vitamin E in lowering the risk for heart disease.

A "Woman Health Study" is evaluating the trial of Vitamin E and beta carotene, and a number of studies are being conducted to check the effectiveness of antioxidants. Fairly strong evidence supports the healthy role of Vitamin E, which along with other antioxidants, are thought to protect body cells from the damaging effects of the so-called oxygen free radicals produced during the body's natural chemical process.

No one contests the statement that most of the United States population would benefit from eating more antioxidant rich food. The question remains: Do the supplementary antioxidants offer any help? This is a controversy for which there is no easy answer. I think that with regular exercise, controlled weight and a healthy diet one should still take extra Vitamin E and C just as an insurance policy in our stressful and polluted world.

Evidence from different studies now indicates that by increasing Vitamin E intake, we can lower our risk of coronary artery disease. In a recent study, about 56 middle-aged people who took vitamin E supplements had markedly less buildup of plaque in their neck arteries compared to those who were not taking the supplements.

I feel strongly that in the near future we will be evaluating the plasma level of antioxidants Vitamin C, E, and beta carotene along with the Homosystine levels, in every patient who has high blood pressure, diabetes and has abnormal lipoprotein and high LP(a) for the risk evaluation of coronary artery disease.

It is appropriate for the patient at risk of coronary artery disease to take Vitamin E supplements and other antioxidants which are plentiful in fruits and vegetables. I recommend 500 mg of Vitamin C daily. The body cannot make Vitamin E, and it is found only in fats and oils; therefore, if you are on a low-fat diet, you must take a Vitamin E supplement of about 400 international units a day, particularly if you have risk of coronary artery disease or if you have diabetes.

Phytochemicals

For hundreds of thousands of years the human race has survived largely on a plant-based diet. Our cells and organs are genetically adapted to that diet. Today, our diet has changed and our drive for material wealth has created more stress in our body and society. Half of the calories we consume in Western society come from animal fat, and that is why we are facing this modern plague of heart disease and cancer.

What are phytochemicals? I consider them to be compounds which fight chemicals causing cancer and heart disease. These natural chemicals are found only in plants. The list of beneficial phytochemicals is growing rapidly. The goal is to develop designer foods or specific fighter chemicals which treat and prevent specific disease.

Black and green tea may contain free radical scavengers. Antioxidants found in India, such as curry powder, garlic, and turmeric are cardio-protective. Other spices and herbs including rosemary, ginger, and sesame seeds, also have antioxidant effects.

Homocystine is another risk factor which recently has been studied extensively. High levels of homocysteine may increase the risk factor for coronary artery disease, and the treatment is fortunately very simple. Just take 1 mg. a day of folic acid and 100 mg of Vitamin B6, and that should take care of it. However, the blood test for homocystein is so costly that for the price of taking the test, you could buy two to three years' supply of folic acid from the store.

Fish oil is known to reduce levels of triglycerides, a major type of fat circulating in the blood. Fish oil contains large amounts of polyunsaturated fatty acids, particularly Omega 3, which fish get from plankton, especially plankton growing in cold water. The most common types of Omega 3 in fish are called EPA or Eicosapentenoic Acid and DHA (Docosahexenoic Acid). When humans eat fatty fish, these Omega 3, working like aspirin, make the platelets in the blood less likely to stick together and also reduce the inflammatory process of the blood vessels. Thus they reduce blood clotting and plaque buildup in the arteries, in turn decreasing the chance of heart attack due clogged coronary arteries.

Perhaps this is why the Japanese and Eskimos, whose diet is heavy in fatty fish, have a low incidence of coronary artery disease. We are not sure if a fish oil supplement is better than eating fish. We do know that if you are taking a supplemental fish oil, prolonged consumption may result in a Vitamin E deficiency because polyunsaturated fat increases the need for vitamin E. So if you are taking fish oil supplements, I recommend also taking vitamin E.

Antioxidants are clearly very important to human life, but they are not elixirs of life. According to scientific findings, your priority should be to improve your lifestyle by eating proper foods and taking antioxidants in the form of vitamins and phytochemicals from fresh fruits and vegetables.

RECOMMENDATIONS:

Eat plenty of fresh fruits and vegetables—at least four to five servings a day.

Decrease your intake of red meat and saturated fats.

Take between 200 to 400 milligrams of Vitamin E (D-Alpha-Tocopherol, *not* DL-Alpha-Tocopherol) from a reliable store. Take these supplements with food as you need fat to absorb and transport the Vitamin E.

Take about 500 milligrams of vitamin C a day, again, from a good supplier. If you cannot eat plenty of fruits and vegetables, then supplement your diet with more Vitamin C.

If you are smoking, *STOP SMOKING* right now!

As our understanding of diet increases, we are learning more about its effect on the human body and how proper diet protects us against disease. Returning to a plant-based diet is the best thing we can do for this human race to survive the next millennium.

12

Vegetarianism

"To be or not to be, that is the question"
—Shakespeare.

IF YOU HAVE A HISTORY OF HEART DISEASE OR
want to prevent having one, let food be your medicine.

Just a few years ago being a vegetarian was anything
but mainstream. Now any time you pick up a leading pub-
lication in a store you will find articles claiming the benefits of being a vegetarian. For the last twenty years scientists all over the world have found that people who
eat more vegetables and fruits have low incidence of heart
disease and cancer. "The Chinese diet study" by Dr. T.
Colin Campbell, a biochemist at Cornell University, found
growing evidence of a link between an animal-based diet
and a wide range of chronic diseases such as heart disease, cancer and osteoporosis.

Dr. Dean Ornish's program for reversing heart disease by lifestyle changes and vegetarian diet has given a new meaning to treatment of heart disease. The Monica study in Europe showed that people consuming more fresh fruits and vegetables (such as in France and Southern Italy) actually had lower incidence of heart disease although the intake of the fat was the same. A Seventh-day Adventist study found that being vegetarian decreases their risk of heart attack.

According to Dr. T. Colin Campbell, early puberty is related to a ten percent higher risk of breast cancer. The World Health Organization has for many year gathered statistics on the age of puberty worldwide. In 1840, the average age of puberty of girls in Western countries was 17, but now it is 12.5. The most likely explanation has to do with diet. Puberty in girls depends on estrogen, a female sex hormone. Meat, poultry and fried food increase estrogen. One way of getting rid of this estrogen is through our digestive tract. The liver alters the estrogen chemically and sends it down to the intestine through bile duct. Fibers from the vegetables and fruits will help the body eliminates the by-product. The American dietary intake of fiber is low and without adequate fibers in the digestive tract the estrogen is reabsorbed into the blood, becoming biologically active.

Estradiol, like testosterone, is carried around the body by a special carrier known as sex-hormone-binding globulin, which keeps them inactive till the body needs them. The soybean contains a natural estrogen known as phtoestrogens which is a weak estrogen that blunts the effect of body estrogen. Researchers have concluded that early puberty may cause cancer in organs that are sensitive to sex hormones such as the breasts.

Our body maintains its daily activity by natural hygienic means. There is a constant tissue building up (anabolism) and tissue breaking down (catabolism) going on in our body by the one trillion cells in our body. In fact three to eight billion of our cells are replaced by new cells every minute. Toxic cells must be removed from your body as soon as possible by a channel of elimination such as the bowel, bladder, lungs and skin. To aid this process of elimination, you must consume more fresh fruits and vegetables.

Our body is made of 70 percent water and 30 percent bones and muscles. Our planet is made of 70 percent water and 30 percent land. If just so happens that to prevent chronic diseases we must consume diet which is 70 percent water and 30 percent solid. The only foods that have a high water content are fresh fruits and vegetables. The rest of our diet should be bread, grain, legumes and dairy products.

In 1973 *The National Geographic* featured a story by a scientist named Alexander Leaf. Dr. Leaf went in search of the oldest people in the world. He found three consistently long-living peoples: the Abkhazians of Russia, the Vilcambans of Ecuador and the Hunzukuts of Pakistan. Not only were these people disease free, but they also had no cancer, no heart disease and were physically active at the age of 100. Dr. Leaf's observation about diet was that all of them were eating food with 70 to 80 percent water content.

Are human beings intended to eat meat?

Consider some of the differences between carnivores (meat-eating animals) and human beings.

Carnivores have long, sharp and pointed teeth. Their jaw moves up and down only. Our teeth are smooth, and our jaw can move from side to side. The saliva of a carnivore is acidic, and the stomach secretes 10 times more hydrochloric acid than does the human stomach. A carnivore's intestine is about three times the length of its trunk so that unused food can be expelled rapidly. Ours is 12 times the length of our trunk and is designed to keep the food in them until all nutrients are extracted. The liver of carnivores can eliminate 10 to 15 times more uric acid than we can. The uric acid is released into our bodies when we consume meat, and we don't have the enzyme uricase to break down uric acid.

Usually there is a concern about protein deficiency for people trying to be vegetarian. That actually is the least of the worries. This issue has been blown out of proportion. A voluminous amount of information shows a direct relationship between high protein foods and heart disease, cancer and other chronic diseases. The association people make between eating meat and providing protein for the body is not based on reality. The body cannot use or assimilate protein as it is eaten. Ingested protein has to be digested and broken down into amino acids. The value of protein in nourishing the body lies in these essential amino acids. There are 23 different amino acids, all of them are needed by the body. Fifteen of them can be produced in the body and the remaining eight must be derived from the food we eat, which is why we call them "essential."

These essential amino acids are available in natural fruits and vegetables including nuts ,seeds and sprouts. Elephants are vegetarian as are camels, mules and water buffalo. If they don't have to eat meat protein for strength, why do we?

It is not easy to change the concept which has been believed for so many years. I don't expect people to become vegetarian overnight, which is why I take a very subtle approach. I believe in educating people with the facts. The rest depends on the individual. If it makes sense to people, they'll change, and if it doesn't they won't.

In late 1970s the incidence of breast cancer in the US was in one out of eleven women and now it is one in eight women. In Japan in the late 1940s breast cancer was rare because Japanese women were consuming only 7 percent of their calories from fat. Now the affluent Japanese who consume more red meat are about 9 times more likely to have breast cancer than are vegetarians.

I think the data is pretty convincing that the vegetarian diet has a healthy edge over a meat diet. We send our kids to the best schools and try to equip them with good values, but we still feed them a diet high in fat that leads to three out of four deaths in our society.

Our body is a beautiful God-given gift, and it is our re-sponsibility to take care of it. If you stop and think of the marvels that our body performs, you will be amazed. Our body takes care of us by self-cleansing, self-healing and self-maintaining itself. It actually is a self-sustained unit by it-self. We experience problems of ill health when we break the laws of nature. The human body is the finest creation; its intelligence is unmatched in power, capacity and adapt-ability.

The body's capacity is mind boggling. The heart has the capability of working nonstop without skipping, pumping 6,300 gallons of blood every day for years and years. Seven million new blood cells are produced every second. And on the top of it, by using the most comprehensive cooling sys-tem in the world with four million pores in the skin, the body maintains an ideal body temperature of 98.6 degrees. Brain cells perform the most tedious jobs, which an advanced computer cannot begin to duplicate. We have trillions of cells which cannot be seen by a human eye without the aid of a microscope. These cells show what is going on inside the cell, the performing of more chemical reactions than all the chemical factories in the world. All the functions of DNA, mitochondria, enzymes and hormones are performing reac-tions that no one on this planet can explain or understand. All this is self-operated by the cells by hygienically balancing the cleansing, healing and maintaining of healthful living. To help our cells perform these marvelous tasks for us, we need to provide the cells of our body with healthy natural nourishment: fruits, vegetables, legumes and other natural foods and food products.

The good news is that more people are taking care of themselves with a vegetarian diet. In 1985, 6.5 million Americans considered themselves to be vegetarian. Six years later, in 1992, nearly twice as many, 12.4 million Ameri-cans, identify themselves as vegetarian. There are four type of vegetarians:

1. Semi Vegetarian: Occasional use of animal product.

2. Ovo-Lacto-Vegetarian: Eats milk products and eggs, avoids meat fish and poultry.

3. Lacto-Vegetarian: Eats milk products, avoids meat, fish, poultry and eggs.

4. Vegetarian (Vegan) Complete vegetarian, avoids animal and dairy products and eggs.

Commonly asked questions about a vegetarian diet

1. Can I get enough protein on a vegetarian diet?

The reality is that our society is getting too much protein. Vegans get 50 to 60 grams of protein a day. Lacto-ovo-vegetarians get 70 to 90 grams of protein a day. The recommended RDA protein allowance is 0.36 grams/pound body weight, or about 43 grams of protein a day for a 120-pound woman. If you are eating enough beans and other vegetable protein, you do not need to worry about this. *Beans have as much protein as beef.* Only severe alcoholics who don't eat for days at a time need to worry about this.

2. Will I shrink my kids if they are on vegetarian diet?

No, they will not look weak, skinny or lack muscle tone. They will not be short of proteins either. I know this from personal experience. If vegetarians look thinner I think it's because the rest of us are overweight.

3. Can I get enough iron?

Yes, by eating dark green leafy vegetables, iron-fortified breads and cereals, dried beans, dried fruit, prune juice, pumpkin seeds, soybeans and nuts. Foods that are high in Vitamin C such as broccoli, tomatoes and green peppers will help the body absorb iron from plant sources.

4. Can I get enough calcium and zinc?

This should not be of any concern. Vegans have better calcium and zinc from plant food. Vegetarians actually absorb and retain calcium better. They also have a lower rate of osteoporosis than meat eaters. Mustard, broccoli, tomatoes and green pepper are good sources of calcium.

5. Do I need to take extra vitamins on a vegetarian diet?

If you are eating enough whole grain foods, wheat germ, spinach, broccoli, and cantaloupe you are consuming enough Vitamin A, C, E, folate and B6. If you want to take an extra precaution you can take Vitamin B12.

6. Are vegeburgers in a restaurant a good choice?

The main ingredients in a vegeburger are soybean, rice and chopped vegetables. Fat content may vary from three to 12 grams; otherwise it is a very good choice. Try different varieties of vegeburgers before deciding if you like them or not. The taste of vegeburgers can vary widely depending on how they are made.

7. Can my family and children eat a vegetarian diet?

It actually may be easier if the whole family adopts the same way of eating. Make sure you eat a balanced diet and keep kids and adults away from nutritionally "empty" foods such as potato chips or candy that can cause dietary deficiencies if they replace nutrient-rich vegetables, fruit, nuts and grains.

8. Is a vegetarian diet tasty? Or do I have to buy exotic foods?

The vegetarian diet can be as tasty as a meat-based diet. You don't have to worry about exotic foods unless you think that pinto beans, cornbread and fruits are exotic!

9. Can I follow a vegetarian diet when I'm eating my meals away from home? What if I can't follow the diet 100 percent?

Most restaurants today try to cater to all of their consumers and offer healthy and tasty vegetarian food. Gone are the days when a vegetarian diet meant broiled vegetables only. My best bet is eating in Chinese, Indian, Italian and Mexican restaurants where the main dishes are vegetarian or can be served without meat. Chefs now take extra effort to present a pleasing and healthy vegetarian meal.

10. Is a vegetarian diet safe?

The answer is simple resounding YES! There is no demonstrable risk to your physical or mental well being from following a vegetarian diet.

Tips on starting on a vegetarian diet

To ease yourself into a vegetarian lifestyle, follow these suggestions:

1. **No more red meat.**

2. **Don't consume more then 6 ounces (the size of a deck of cards) of fish and or poultry a day.**

3. **Start having at least one or two meatless meal a week.**

4. **Start eliminating butter and animal-based**

oils for your favorite recipes and start substituting margarine and low-fat mayonnaise and oils.

5. Increase the use of tofu, nonfat yogurt and applesauce.

6. Eat more fresh fruits and vegetables.

After a few weeks. . .

1. Decrease the portion of fish and poultry to 3 ounces a day.

2. Try to have about four meatless meals a week.

3. Try different beans and pasta combinations, and bean soup.

4. Be bold enough to try different vegetarian recipes from different cook books.

5. Once you willingly convince yourself why you are accepting food as medicine for your mind and body you will feel more connected with yourself.

Continue these suggestions till you get rid of the meat completely. Of course, an even better choice if you can muster the will power is simply to plunge into the new way of eating and become an instant vegetarian.

Being a vegetarian does not make you a "health nut," but a "health smart" person. Remember that your body is meticulously working for you to maintain vital functions. By providing the proper nourishment to your body's cells you not only add years to your life but also avoid chronic diseases and won't allow your "golden years of life" to be "wasting years of life" spent shuttling between the doctor's office and the prescription counter.

Vegetarianism is not a cult but a necessity for heart healthy living.

Fat Percentage Calculator

Grams of fat	1	2	3	4	5	6	7	8	9	10	11	12	13	14	15	16	17
Calories																	
25	36%	72%															
50	18%	36%	54%	72%	90%												
75	12%	24%	36%	48%	60%	72%	84%	96%									
100	9%	18%	27%	36%	45%	54%	63%	72%	81%	90%	99%						
125	7%	14%	22%	29%	36%	43%	50%	58%	65%	72%	79%	86%	94%				
150	6%	12%	18%	24%	30%	36%	42%	48%	54%	60%	66%	72%	78%	84%	91%	96%	
175	5%	10%	15%	21%	26%	31%	36%	41%	46%	51%	57%	62%	67%	72%	77%	82%	87%
200	5%	9%	14%	18%	23%	27%	32%	36%	41%	45%	50%	54%	59%	63%	68%	72%	77%
225	4%	8%	12%	16%	20%	24%	28%	32%	36%	40%	44%	48%	52%	56%	60%	64%	68%
250	4%	7%	11%	14%	18%	22%	25%	29%	32%	36%	40%	44%	48%	52%	56%	60%	64%
275	3%	7%	10%	13%	16%	20%	23%	26%	29%	33%	36%	39%	43%	46%	49%	52%	56%
300	3%	6%	9%	12%	15%	18%	21%	24%	27%	30%	33%	36%	39%	42%	45%	48%	51%
325	3%	6%	8%	11%	14%	17%	19%	22%	25%	28%	30%	33%	36%	39%	42%	44%	47%
350	3%	5%	8%	10%	13%	15%	18%	21%	23%	26%	28%	31%	33%	36%	39%	41%	44%
375	2%	5%	7%	10%	12%	14%	17%	19%	22%	24%	26%	29%	31%	34%	36%	38%	41%
400	2%	5%	7%	9%	11%	14%	16%	18%	20%	23%	25%	27%	29%	31%	34%	36%	38%

13

Drug Treatment

IN THE PAST DECADE WE HAVE SEEN A MAJOR
shift in the management of high cholesterol. Trials of HMG-
CoA reductase inhibitors indicate that by reducing cholesterol we can offer a greater protection against coronary artery disease. One out of three Americans adults has a cholesterol level of more then 240. Although cholesterol is only
one of the multiple risk factors for coronary artery disease,
there is no longer any doubt that lowering cholesterol, particularly LDL cholesterol, will reduce the mortality and mor-
bidity from coronary artery disease.

Before you start taking medication for high cholesterol,
keep in mind that you can lower your total cholesterol by
lifestyle changes alone, especially by modifying your diet by
restricting use of saturated fats and cholesterol. As with all
medications, cholesterol-lowering medications should be
prescribed with restraint. Their use to treat lipid disorders

should be considered as an adjunct to diet, only after all probable causes have been excluded or treated, and after dietary modification has been given an adequate trial.

In my practice, I have seen many patients taking these medications and complaining that they are not helping them reduce their cholesterol levels as much as expected. The truth is that medication is just part of the whole treatment plan. These HMG-CoA reductase inhibitors are powerful drugs and should be taken properly. All the other lifestyle changes such as exercising, eating a low-fat diet and reducing stress should be exhausted before starting on these medications. If you do all of these, then medication can complement the holistic treatment plan to achieve your target, which is decreasing the LDL (bad) cholesterol.

As I have discussed before, a low-fat low-cholesterol diet is a cornerstone for the treatment of lipid disorders. You do not need to be an expert on nutrition; the only thing you need to know is how to calculate the percentage of fat and fat calories in food. In addition, it would be a good idea to increase your intake of fiber. You need to consume about twenty grams of fiber a day. You should exercise about twenty to thirty minutes a day, and you should give at least three to six months for your diet to work before jumping into medications.

The decision about how to manage cholesterol is governed by whether your goal is primary or secondary prevention. Primary prevention includes persons who have never had heart disease but are perceived to be at high risk. Secondary prevention applies to patients who already have coronary artery disease.

Half of the patients admitted to hospitals with angina or acute MI may have cholesterol levels of about 200. We know that to prevent atherosclerosis the total cholesterol level should be 180 or lower. Actually for the last five or ten years many studies have been done to substantiate this claim, such as those by the National Health Lung and Blood Institute, a lipid research clinic primary prevention trial, the Helsinki health study, the "Four S "study and recently a primary prevention trial in west Scotland. All of these studies confirm the hypothesis that lowering bad cholesterol (LDL) not only reduces the risk of coronary artery disease but also stops its progression and in some cases reverses the atherosclerosis. All of them basically convey the same message: drug therapy prescribed for an adequate length of time, complemented by proper diet, exercise and stress management, will not only stop coronary artery disease (Primary Prevention), but will also help in the reversal of coronary artery disease (Secondary Prevention).

First Line Agents:

The two first-line agents in lowering cholesterol are (1) bile acid raisin and (2) nicotinic acid.

Bile acid-binding raisins also have some side effects, such as constipation or bloating, and may lead to more absorption of fat and other side effects in the digestive system. These side effects have displeased many physicians and patients. Manufacturers have tried to improve the situation by making the medicine in the form of tablets and bars, but their results have not been very successful.

The second drug is nicotinic acid or niacin. This drug has been used to lower cholesterol since 1955. It has the beneficial effect of decreasing bad cholesterol (LDL), and raising good cholesterol (HDL). Unfortunately, it has very unpleasant side effects such as flushing of the face and body, itching, stomach upset, and gastric irritation. Rarely, it can damage the liver. If you have high blood sugar, niacin may increase the level of your blood sugar and can also make gout symptoms worse by increasing blood uric acid. To be effective as a drug, niacin has to be taken in high doses. At the mega dose level, niacin is potentially hazardous and should be taken only under physician supervision in order to monitor the liver function. Sustained release or long-acting niacin should not be taken. You should start with a very low dose of 50 mg. once a day and slowly increase that to about 1500 mg. a day. I have used this prescription aggressively for patients who are young if they also have a high

Lp(a), another type of cholesterol which presently can be treated only by high-dose niacin.

Second Line Agents:

1. Probucol

This drug is not used much, because it reduces the good cholesterol (HDL) along with total cholesterol.

2. Gemfibrozil

Gemfibrozil is a safe and effective triglyceride-lowering drug. It also increases the HDL and reduces the incidence of coronary disease. The major drawback is that it is ineffective in reducing overall cholesterol and LDL cholesterol. It has been used in association with HMG CoA Reductase Inhibitors.

3. HMG-CoA Reductase Inhibitors

These agents were approved for use in the United States in the early 1990s for the treatment of high cholesterol which is unresponsive to diet therapy. It is a substantially more effective LDL cholesterol reduction agent than the bile acid or bile acid and niacin combined. The HMG-CoA Reductase Inhibitors are prescribed to be taken one a day and have minimal side effects. Three agents—lovastatin, simastatin and pravastatin—have attained approval for use in the United States. Atorvastatin, a newer HMG-CoA Reductase Inhibitor is not at this writing available for clinical use in the US.

These HMG-CoA Reductase Inhibitors are extremely effective and could decrease an individual's LDL by 20 to 45 percent, increase HDL by about 10 percent, and decrease triglycerides by about 20 to 25 percent. Reduction varies with every medication, but on average, this drug can effectively lower the cholesterol, particularly total cholesterol and bad cholesterol (LDL)

As a general rule, a small dose of medication is given at bedtime and cholesterol and liver enzymes are checked every two or three months until target cholesterol levels have been achieved, however, the liver enzymes and cholesterol is checked every six months.

New research findings continue to enrich our knowledge about lipoprotein complexity and particularly how to treat cholesterol abnormalities. With the present knowledge that we have, I strongly advise all patients that drug therapy should never be a sole treatment. It has to be complemented with life style changes to ensure success.

Reversal of Heart Disease
Comparison of Programs

	Ornish	Schuler	Saini
Calories from fat	10%	20%	15%
Aerobic exercise	3 hrs/ week	30 min/ day	3 hrs/ week
Stress management	1 hr/ day	Recommended	1/2 hr/ day
Support group	2 hrs/ week	1 hr/ day	Recommended

Finally. . .

ALL MEN AND WOMEN MAKE MISTAKES, BUT all wise men and women are less apt to make them the second time. Through the process of learning from our mistakes, we can have a brighter expectation tomorrow. This is reason enough for living.

No matter what you have acquired—wealth, education or prestige—ask yourself if you are happier, wiser and healthier. If not, then explore the cause in your heart. You will find that it is largely an internal problem. Look within you to see if you need to develop self control for your impulsiveness. The answer is within you.

In this book I have mentioned repeatedly (nine times) the role of stressors in coronary artery disease. I have mentioned that for two out of three of our patients who have joined the cardiac rehab program, the major cause of the disease is the toxic stress. All other risk factors are secondary to the person's psychological profile. If you are impulsive, resistant to change, and isolated, your stress and your coping mechanism will override all other information being provided to you. After spending fifteen minutes with the dietitian and fifteen minutes with the physician you will not remember anything which was conveyed to you. This is a waste of time. For such patients it is absolutely imperative for health care practitioners to spend a good deal of time with them to help them realize that their risk factors can be improved but only if they realize that they have to accept this and change their personality and learn how to manage stress first.

It is not only possible to prevent illness through behavioral, dietary, and attitudinal changes, but also to evoke healing from within the body itself. The human body has evolved, over millions of years of evolution, to a package of formidable intelligence. And it is this intelligence that is the ultimate and supreme genius which mirrors the wisdom of the universe.

We know that the body is its own pharmacy. It is capable of making wonder drugs such as tranquilizers, sleeping pills, immuno-modulators, and antihypertensive chemicals to mention a few. In addition, the body makes these chemical substances and delivers them in the right dose to each organ. This is *internal* medicine without side effects and with no need for written instructions.

More people in our civilized world die on Monday than on any other day of the week. Human beings are the only living species that differentiate time. For people with no standard risk factors, the leading cause of coronary disease is not job dissatisfaction but rather the lack of purpose and meaning in life.

Next time if you are stressed out, ask yourself—

"Is it worth dying for?"

If it is not, then let it go so that you can create a healthy heart.

And remember this quote from Michael Pritchard:

"You don't stop laughing because you grow old. You grow old because you stopped laughing."

GLOSSARY

Adrenaline: A secretion of adrenal glands which constricts blood vessels and increases heart rate and blood pressure.

Aerobic Exercise: Physical exercise that relies on oxygen for energy production and therefore can be sustained for a long period of time.

Alcohol: An intoxicating ingredient in beer, wine and hard liquor.

Anaerobic exercise: Physical exercise that does not rely on oxygen for energy production and therefore can be sustained only for a short period of time.

Angina: Temporary pain in the chest caused by the heart muscle when a part of the muscle did not receive enough oxygen rich blood.

Angiogram: An X-ray of the heart and blood vessels after injecting of a dye into the blood stream.

Angioplasty: A technique to dilate the obstructed artery by balloon or other devices.

Aorta: The largest artery of the body, originating from the heart and transports blood to the main arteries.

Arteriole: The smallest type of the artery which transports the blood to the cells.

Arrythmia: Irregular heart beat.

Atherosclerosis: Also known as hardening of the artery; thought to be leading cause of death. In this process of hardening fat, blood clotting materials and calcium builds up inside the inner wall of the arteries causing it to restrict the blood flow to the cells.

Bypass surgery: a surgical technique by which blood is detoured around a blocked artery using vein or an artery from another part of the body.

Calorie: A unit that express the heat or energy value of the food. The only substances that provide calories are carbohydrates, proteins, fat and alcohol.

Cardiovascular: Pertaining to the heart and blood vessels.

Cardiovascular fitness: The ability of the circulatory system to meet the body's demand for physical activity.

Catheter: A thin tube of plastic inserted into a vein or artery and advanced to the heart with X-ray guidance.

Cholesterol: A fat-like waxy substance present in the blood, liver, brain and all other tissues in the body. It is made by the liver and found in food of animal origin.

Collaterals: Blood vessels which branch off from nearby arteries to provide blood to the heart muscle which was not adequately supplied due to the obstruction of the artery.

Coronary: Heart.

Coronary arteries: Arteries which arise from aorta and feed the heart muscle a supply of oxygen-rich blood.

Coronary Artery Disease: Disease of the arteries (atherosclerosis) leading to angina and or heart attack.

Ejection Fraction: Percentage of blood in the left ventricle that is pumped out during each heart beat.

Heart attack: Death of heart muscle caused by a prolonged period of no supply of oxygen to that part of the muscle.

Heart Failure: A condition in which the heart muscle is unable to fully pump the blood out of the heart.

Hypertension: The term used to define a blood pressure which is above the normal range.

Fat: One of the three major source of energy in the food.

Fatty Acid: A chemical unit of fat, saturated and unsaturated.

Fiber: An important part of our diet, more commonly known as roughage. Fiber can be broken down to two categories:

Soluble Fiber: Binds bile salts and cholesterol in the digestive system, hinders the reabsorption of cholesterol and promotes its excretion from the body. That is why high-fiber grains such as oats and rice may lower the serum cholesterol.

Insoluble Fiber: Increases fecal bulk, thereby speeding the food through the stomach and intestines. Insoluble fibers have poor water-holding capacity.

Heart Rate: Number of beats of the heart per minute.

HDL (High Density Lipoprotein): A body chemical that carries and removes cholesterol from the cell and delivers it to the liver for processing.

Hydrogenation: A chemical process which makes fats from saturated fat. During the chemical process it adds hydrogen atoms to the fatty acid.

Hypertension: High blood pressure.

LDL (Low Density Lipoprotein): Like HDL, this is also a carrier for the cholesterol but instead of removing the cholesterol from the cells to be brought to the liver, LDL carriers often lose some of the cholesterol on their way. This cholesterol is deposited in the arterial wall leading to coronary artery disease.

Lipid: Fat.

Lipoprotein: A protein which transports fats through blood stream.

MET (Metabolic Equivalent Unit): a measure of human energy output.

Monounsaturated Fat: A type of fat which is considered to be healthy for you and which does not increase the total cholesterol. It does not decrease the good cholesterol (HDL) either. Common types of monounsaturated oils are canola, olive and peanut oil.

Myocardial Infarction: A medical term that means "Heart Attack."

Myocardial Ischemia: suppression of the flow of blood in the heart.

Platelets: Blood cells that play an important role in the formation of blood clots and plaque.

Polyunsaturated Fat: Usually in the liquid form at room temperature, originates with plants and fish oil. Polyunsaturated fats can lower both the LDL and HDL cholesterol. Common types of oil high in this type of fat are corn, soya bean, cottonseed, sunflower and safflower oil.

Plaque: A buildup of cholesterol and other fatty deposits in an arterial wall.

Saturated Fat: Usually solid at room temperature and comes from both animals and plants. Saturated fats are known as cholesterol boosters because they increase LDL cholesterol. Common examples of saturated fat are butter. lard, meat fat, coconut oil, palm oil and palm-kernel oil.

Thallium Scan (SPECT Thallium): A nuclear stress test by a radioactive isotope which is injected in the vein during exercise and then measured with a special instrument to detect myocardial ischemia.

Triglycerides: A type of fatty substance found in the body which increases with fat, sugar and alcohol intake.

Unstable angina: A worsening of angina which may cause heart attack.

Order Sheet for additional copies

Please send ___ copies of *Create a Healthy Heart* at US$15.00 each plus $3.00 shipping and handling to:

Name: _____

Address: _____

City: _____ State: _____ Zip: _____

Mail this order form to:

     Healthy Heart Publishing
     3135 Imperial Blvd.
     Springfield, OH 45503

Make your check or money order payable to Healthy Heart Publishing.

Ohio residents, add $0.90 sales tax per book.

Order Sheet for additional copies

Please send ___ copies of *Create a Healthy Heart* at US$15.00 each plus $3.00 shipping and handling to:

Name: _____

Address: _____

City: _____ State: _____ Zip: _____

Mail this order form to:

     Healthy Heart Publishing
     3135 Imperial Blvd.
     Springfield, OH 45503

Make your check or money order payable to Healthy Heart Publishing.

Ohio residents, add $0.90 sales tax per book.